KU-606-862

WITHDRAWN FROM STOCK
DUBLIN CITY PUBLIC LIBRARIES

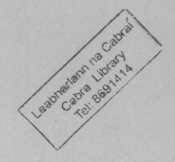
Leabharlann na Cabrai
Cabra Library
Tel: 8691414

DK

BODY MOT

CONTENTS

Introduction   **6**

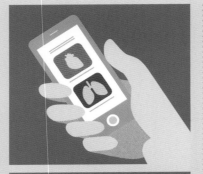

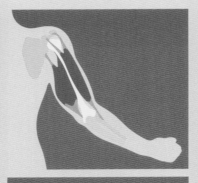

MONITORING YOUR HEALTH

GENERAL ADULT TESTS

Why monitor your health?   **10**

Environmental and personal factors   **12**

Behavioural factors   **14**

Types of health check   **16**

Medical checks   **18**

DIY health checks   **20**

Body weight   **24**

Your heart and circulation   **26**

Measuring blood pressure   **28**

What your blood pressure reading means   **30**

Checking your heart rate   **32**

Measuring your heart's rhythm   **34**

Exercise electrocardiogram   **36**

Echocardiography   **38**

Abdominal aortic aneurysm scan   **40**

How breathing works   **42**

Chest X-ray   **44**

Measuring peak flow   **45**

Spirometry   **46**

Lung volume   **48**

Exercise capacity   **50**

Blood oxygenation   **51**

The roles of blood   **52**

Giving a blood sample   **54**

Blood count   **55**

Checking blood glucose   **56**

Checking blood cholesterol   **58**

Other blood tests   **60**

Checking for allergies   **62**

Your digestive system   **64**

Screening for bowel cancer   **66**

Testing for *H. pylori*   **68**

Abdominal ultrasound   **70**

Liver blood tests   **71**

How your kidneys work   **72**

Urine analysis   **74**

Testing kidney function   **76**

The male reproductive system   **78**

Checking for infections   **80**

Checking the testicles   **82**

Checking the prostate   **83**

The female reproductive system   **84**

Testing for pregnancy   **86**

Checking for infections   **88**

Pelvic examination   **90**

Colposcopy   **91**

Checking for cervical cancer   **92**

 Penguin Random House

DK LONDON

Senior Art Editor
Sharon Spencer

Project Art Editor
Francis Wong

Illustrators
Mark Clifton, Phil Gamble,
Gus Scott

Producer (Pre-production)
Robert Dunn

Senior Producer
Meskerem Berhane

Managing Art Editor
Michael Duffy

Art Director
Karen Self

Senior Editors
Jemima Dunne, Rob Houston,
Martyn Page

Project Editor
Miezan van Zyl

**Jackets Design
Development Manager**
Sophia MTT

Managing Editor
Angeles Gavira Guerrero

**Associate Publishing
Director**
Liz Wheeler

Publishing Director
Jonathan Metcalf

DK INDIA

Project Art Editor
Rupanki Arora Kaushik

Art Editors
Rabia Ahmad, Mridushmita Bose

Assistant Art Editor
Garima Agarwal

Illustrators
Arshti Narang, Anjali Sachar

Managing Art Editor
Sudakshina Basu

DTP Designer
Nityanand Kumar

Pre-production Manager
Balwant Singh

Senior Editor
Dharini Ganesh

Editor
Priyanjali Narain

Senior Managing Editor
Rohan Sinha

Jacket Designer
Priyanka Bansal

Senior DTP Designer
Shanker Prasad

Assistant Picture Researcher
Geetika Bhandari

Picture Research Manager
Taiyaba Khatoon

Production Manager
Pankaj Sharma

Checking for breast cancer   94
Your skin   96
Checking your skin   98
How the eyes work   100
Testing vision   102
Testing for astigmatism   104
Colour vision test   105
Checking your eye health   106
Testing visual field   108
Measuring eye pressure   109
How the ears work   110
Testing your hearing   112
Tympanometry   114
Mouth and teeth   116
Dental check-up   118
Your skeleton   120
Your muscles   122
Flexibility, posture, and gait   124
Core stability testing   126
Muscle strength and endurance   128
Your nervous system   130
How your nervous system works   132
Testing your reflexes   134
Testing coordination and balance   134
Testing sensory nerve pathways   136
How your mind works   138
Mood analysis   140
Dementia testing   140

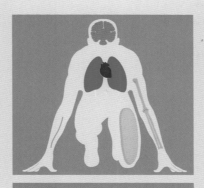

OPTIMIZING YOUR HEALTH

Vaccinations   144
A healthy diet   146
Adapting your diet   148
Alcohol, tobacco, and drugs   150
Keeping fit   152
Exercise for special groups   154
Safeguarding your bones and muscles   156
Keeping your skin healthy   158
Ear health   160
Eye health   161
Sexual health   162
Psychological health   164

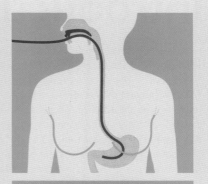

OTHER TESTS AND YOUR RECORDS

Other medical tests   168
Health screening options   176
Vaccination record   178
Weight record   180
Blood pressure record   181
Health checks record   182

Index   184
Acknowledgments   192

First published in Great Britain in 2020
by Dorling Kindersley Limited
80 Strand, London, WC2R 0RL

Copyright © 2020 Dorling Kindersley Limited
A Penguin Random House Company
10 9 8 7 6 5 4 3 2 1
001–314651–Feb/2020

All rights reserved.
No part of this publication may be reproduced, stored in or introduced into a retrieval system, or transmitted, in any form, or by any means (electronic, mechanical, photocopying, recording, or otherwise), without the prior written permission of the copyright owner.

A CIP catalogue record for this book
is available from the British Library.
ISBN: 978-0-2413-8680-4

Printed in China

A WORLD OF IDEAS:
SEE ALL THERE IS TO KNOW

www.dk.com

CONTRIBUTORS

Jess Baker, Mike Blanchard, Dr Michelle Booth, Dr Claudia Brown, Dr Nicola Renton, Kate Crouch, Katie John, Dr Dina Kaufman, Dr Mark Roussot, Dr Erlina Saeed, Dr Simone Shelley, Dr Kate Tuffy, Dr Frances Williams

MEDICAL CONSULTANT

Dr Kristina Routh

READER NOTICE

Body MOT provides information on a wide range of medical topics, and every effort has been made to ensure that the information in this book is accurate and up-to-date (as at the date of publication). The book is not a substitute for expert medical advice, however, and is not to be relied on for medical, healthcare, pharmaceutical, or other professional advice on specific circumstances and in specific locations. You are advised always to consult a doctor or other health professional for specific information on personal health matters. Please consult your GP before changing, stopping, or starting any medical treatment. Never disregard expert medical advice or delay in seeking advice or treatment due to information obtained from this book. The naming of any product, treatment, or organization in this book does not imply endorsement by the consultants, contributors, or publisher, nor does the omission of any such names indicate disapproval. The consultants, contributors, and publisher do not accept any legal responsibility for any personal injury or other damage or loss arising directly or indirectly from any use or misuse of the information and advice in this book.

Introduction

In recent years, there has been a quiet revolution in medicine and healthcare, with a move away from the traditional emphasis on treating disease and increasingly towards prevention. Moreover, the concept of prevention itself has expanded, from simply preventing disease towards actively taking measures to optimize health. Key aspects of this new trend in health maximization are screening tests for particular conditions and regular monitoring of significant indicators of health, such as blood pressure, in order to spot early signs of a potential problem so that it can be dealt with before it develops into illness. Furthermore, with new technology, you can monitor many aspects of your health yourself, so that you can get expert medical advice early. Health professionals also increasingly benefit from new technology to offer a range of sophisticated health checks and tests.

However, the many health check options available can be confusing. This book aims to demystify health screening and tests so that you can make good choices about monitoring and maintaining your health. The book is divided into four main sections. The first, "Monitoring your health", provides an overview of health and health checks, from the factors that affect your health to the ways in which you can keep a check on your health. The second section, "General adult tests", gives detailed, accessible information about the most common and useful tests, including not only tests that a health professional might carry out, but also those you can do yourself, such as checking your skin. The third section, "Optimizing your health", gives practical advice on measures you can take to ensure you keep as healthy as possible, from diet and exercise, to information about vaccinations and psychological health. The final section includes information about important, but less commonly performed medical tests, such as biopsies to analyse tissue samples, as well as an overview of screening options to consider and pages for you to copy and use to record your own and your family's health check results.

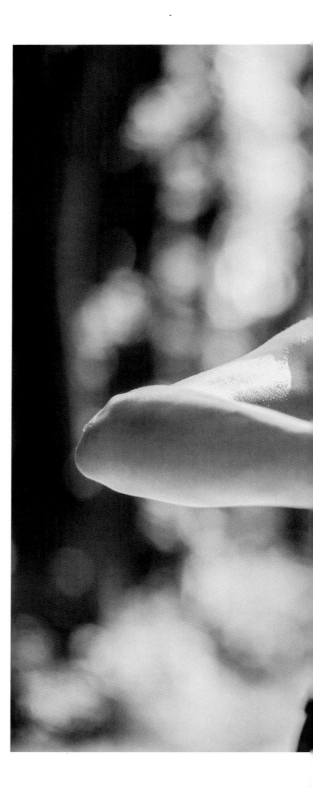

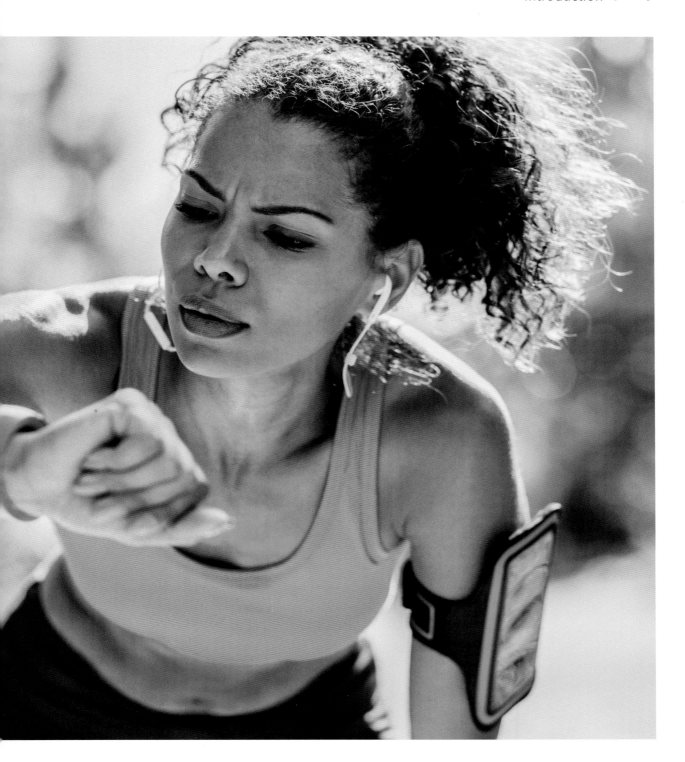

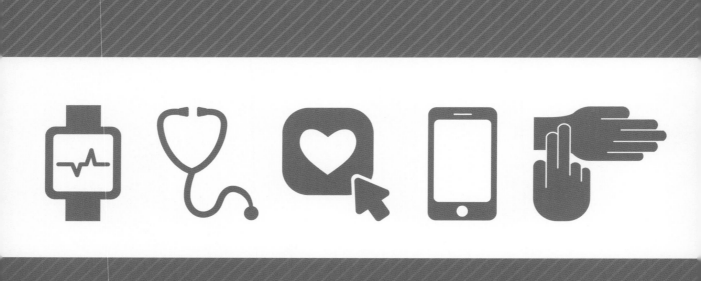

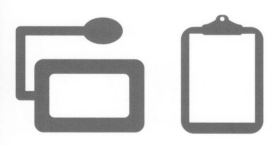

Monitoring your health

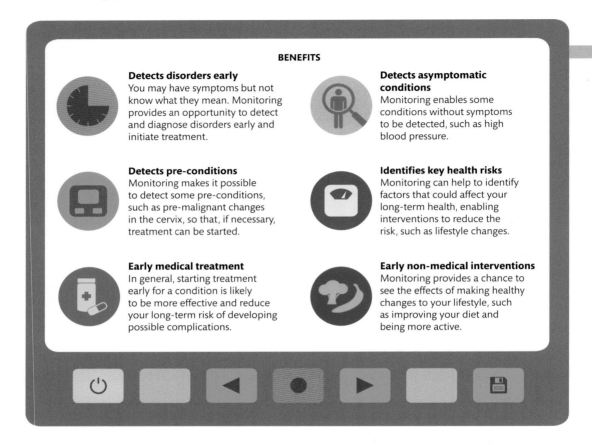

BENEFITS

Detects disorders early
You may have symptoms but not know what they mean. Monitoring provides an opportunity to detect and diagnose disorders early and initiate treatment.

Detects asymptomatic conditions
Monitoring enables some conditions without symptoms to be detected, such as high blood pressure.

Detects pre-conditions
Monitoring makes it possible to detect some pre-conditions, such as pre-malignant changes in the cervix, so that, if necessary, treatment can be started.

Identifies key health risks
Monitoring can help to identify factors that could affect your long-term health, enabling interventions to reduce the risk, such as lifestyle changes.

Early medical treatment
In general, starting treatment early for a condition is likely to be more effective and reduce your long-term risk of developing possible complications.

Early non-medical interventions
Monitoring provides a chance to see the effects of making healthy changes to your lifestyle, such as improving your diet and being more active.

Why monitor your health?

Health is a state of physical and mental wellbeing and not merely the absence of disease. Generally, most people are well most of the time. However, health monitoring is useful because it can detect risk factors or the early signs of a condition that might become a health problem.

Advantages and disadvantages of monitoring
Monitoring provides a positive way for you to learn about your own body, and is an opportunity for you to engage with and affect your own health. Early detection of conditions by monitoring can even improve your life expectancy. For example, by detecting pre-diabetes, early medical intervention together with lifestyle changes could delay the onset of the disease itself by several years.

However, it is important that monitoring provides accurate results that do not lead to unnecessary further tests because of a wrong positive result or lead to you ignoring symptoms because of a wrong negative result. Although health monitoring tests are not perfect, in general, monitoring is beneficial because of the advantage of early identification of a problem, and because identifying risk factors early may help you take appropriate action.

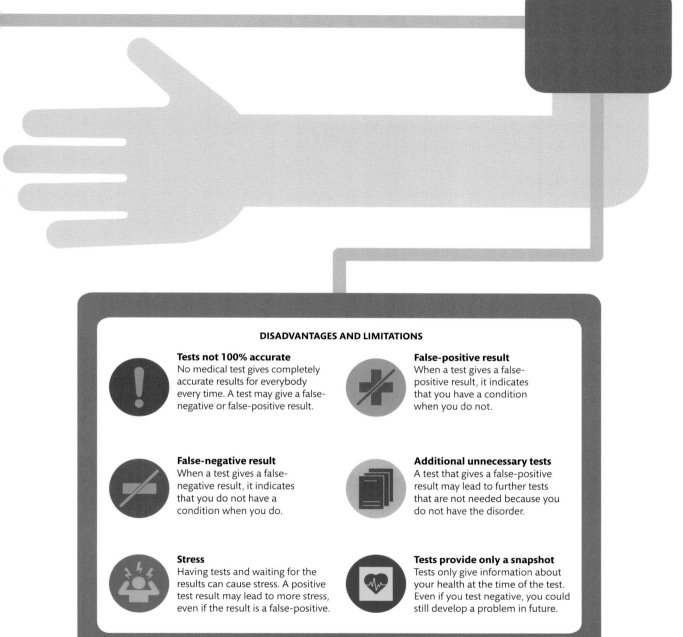

DISADVANTAGES AND LIMITATIONS

Tests not 100% accurate
No medical test gives completely accurate results for everybody every time. A test may give a false-negative or false-positive result.

False-positive result
When a test gives a false-positive result, it indicates that you have a condition when you do not.

False-negative result
When a test gives a false-negative result, it indicates that you do not have a condition when you do.

Additional unnecessary tests
A test that gives a false-positive result may lead to further tests that are not needed because you do not have the disorder.

Stress
Having tests and waiting for the results can cause stress. A positive test result may lead to more stress, even if the result is a false-positive.

Tests provide only a snapshot
Tests only give information about your health at the time of the test. Even if you test negative, you could still develop a problem in future.

Environmental and personal factors

A wide range of factors affect your health. Some of these are outside your control, including environmental factors, such as a safe water supply and clean air, and personal factors such as your age, gender, and genetic inheritance.

Environmental factors

Your physical environment plays an important role in your quality of health. It determines your exposure to physical, biological, and chemical agents that might affect your health, such as hazardous substances that could be ingested, inhaled, or absorbed through the skin. Not only can a healthy environment reduce the likelihood of health problems, it can also increase your lifespan.

Safe water
Clean drinking water and good sanitation are important in reducing the risk of water-borne infections and exposure to harmful chemicals that may affect us and the food we eat.

Clean air
Pollution-free air, both inside and outside the home, can significantly reduce the chance of developing respiratory diseases.

Good housing
Good housing helps to reduce the spread of infections and minimizes exposure to hazardous materials.

Good public transport
A good public transport system can lead to reduced car usage and lower pollution. Having better pavements, cycle lanes, and trails encourages physical activity.

Healthy workplace
Good working practices reduce exposure to unsafe environments. They also minimize the risk of occupational disorders.

Good social services
Accessible, high-quality social services, such as health services, can ensure that fundamental needs are met, which is especially important for those with special health needs.

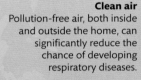
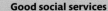

Personal factors

As well as environmental factors, your health is also significantly influenced by a wide range of factors individual to you. Many of these factors depend on your parents; for example, your genetic inheritance, ethnicity, and family medical history. Your family, together with your peers, also influence your health in more subtle ways, by influencing behaviour, for example (see pp.14–15).

Age

In general, health declines with age. As you age, it is important to exercise and eat healthily. You should stay in touch with friends and family and look after your mental and physical health.

Genetics

The genes you inherit from your parents determine many characteristics, from hair colour to susceptibility to various diseases. In some cases, a gene may mutate and cause disease.

Gender

On average, women live longer than men. Men and women also tend to suffer from different illnesses. For example, men can develop prostate cancer and women can develop gynaecological cancers.

Ethnicity

Ethnicity plays a large role in your wellbeing. It influences your culture, lifestyle, and customs. These, in turn, influence your diet and habits such as smoking, and can make you more prone to certain illnesses, such as diabetes.

Family medical history

Some conditions tend to run in families, such as asthma and heart disease. Knowing your family medical history can help identify possible health problems and enable you to take measures to reduce risk factors.

Personal medical history

Your medical history – for example, immunizations, illnesses, and medication – can not only affect your present health but may also influence future wellbeing by affecting your risk of developing various disorders.

Weight

It is important to maintain a healthy weight to maximize health. Body shape is also important: a large amount of fat around your abdomen is worse for your health than fat around your thighs and buttocks.

Height

It is not clear how height affects health but, on average, tall people have a lower chance of developing heart disease and dementia but a higher risk of certain cancers than shorter people.

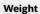

Behavioural factors

In addition to personal and environmental factors (see pp.12–13), behavioural factors also influence your health. Furthermore, behavioural factors are largely within your control – you can choose what to eat and how much exercise to do, for example – and so you can actively choose to improve your health.

Diet
A healthy diet can reduce your risk of obesity and of certain diseases, such as diabetes. Eating plenty of vegetables, fruit, and fibre, using unsaturated fats, and eating low-fat protein can maximize your health.

Exercise
Regular exercise improves the quality of life, enhances mental wellbeing, and increases life expectancy. To benefit your health, every week aim to do at least 150 minutes of exercise that raises your heart rate.

Smoking
If you smoke, stopping is probably the most important thing you can do to improve your health. It is never too late to stop, but the sooner you stop, the greater the reduction in your risk of smoking-related diseases.

Drug use
It is important to take medication only as advised by a healthcare professional. Recreational drug use can severely damage physical and mental health, and can be fatal. It can also affect relationships and work life.

Alcohol use
Excessive alcohol use can seriously damage your health, and the more you drink, the greater the health risk. However, drinking a small amount may help to protect against heart disease and stroke.

Sleep
Most adults need seven to nine hours of sleep a night. Good sleep improves concentration, motivation, and mood. Exercise, reducing the time using a computer, and cutting down alcohol intake can help to improve sleep.

Behaviour, lifestyle, and health

Your lifestyle can have a large impact on your health. To some extent, lifestyle behaviours are influenced by your family and peers; for example, if they generally follow a healthy lifestyle, such as exercising regularly and not smoking or using recreational drugs, you are also likely to do the same. However, ultimately it is your personal choice about which lifestyle behaviours to adopt.

Relationships

Good-quality relationships with family, friends, and the community in which you live are important for both your physical and mental wellbeing, helping you to have a longer, happier life with fewer mental-health issues.

Social life and leisure

An active social life and engaging in leisure activities can help to reduce stress and improve physical and mental wellbeing. Social isolation is linked with higher rates of illness and decreased life satisfaction.

Sexual health

Safer-sex methods reduce your risk of catching a sexually transmitted infection. For heterosexual sex, they also reduce the likelihood of an unwanted pregnancy. The fewer partners you have, the lower the risk of catching an STI.

Occupation

A good-quality job, with adequate pay, protection from physical hazards, job security, and job satisfaction, is associated with a higher level of both physical and psychological wellbeing.

Stress

In the short term, a certain amount of stress can be positive because it can help to motivate you. However, long-term stress can damage your physical health and cause anxiety and depression.

Income

For reasons that are not entirely clear, people with higher incomes are generally less at risk from mental illness, harm from drugs, alcohol, or smoking, and from emotional issues.

Types of health check

There are a range of health checks available, from those carried out by your own doctor, to workplace assessments, and specific tests required by certain occupations or organizations. The aim is to identify those at risk of specific medical conditions and/or ensure people meet safety standards required to carry out a particular job. Checks not only include medical tests by health professionals (see pp.18–19), you can also monitor your own health at home and online (see pp.20–21).

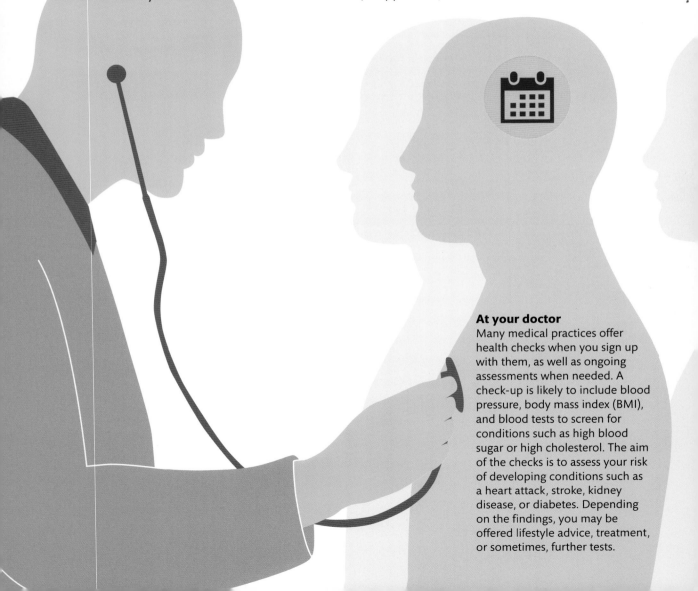

At your doctor
Many medical practices offer health checks when you sign up with them, as well as ongoing assessments when needed. A check-up is likely to include blood pressure, body mass index (BMI), and blood tests to screen for conditions such as high blood sugar or high cholesterol. The aim of the checks is to assess your risk of developing conditions such as a heart attack, stroke, kidney disease, or diabetes. Depending on the findings, you may be offered lifestyle advice, treatment, or sometimes, further tests.

PREPARING FOR A MEDICAL

You do not need to do much preparation as health assessments aim to evaluate your baseline health status, but gathering some background information will help your doctor.

- Find out about the medical history of your immediate family, particularly for any conditions such as strokes, heart attacks, diabetes, or high cholesterol, as well as cancers, including their ages at diagnosis.
- Take a list of the medications you take regularly, including those bought over the counter, such as pain relief, vitamin and mineral supplements, as well as non-medical preparations.
- Make a note of any known intolerances or allergies.
- Bring a list of vaccinations you have been given, and when you had them.
- Write down your own concerns or questions you want to ask the health professional, about links to family medical history, for example.

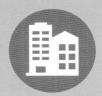

Workplace health checks

Many companies offer medical check-ups when you join, as well as ongoing health monitoring. These usually comprise similar assessments to those carried out by your doctor, and if they identify abnormalities, they will usually refer you to your doctor. Some professions have further checks as a requirement for employment. For example, bus or train drivers need to undergo regular fit-to-work assessments. Commercial pilots must have a medical certificate that needs updating regularly.

Other health checks

Health checks may be requested by external organizations, too. Sports bodies require athletes to undergo cardiology screening and tests for performance- enhancing drugs before they can compete. Private medical and life insurance companies may ask you to have a medical before signing up for a policy. When you join a gym or enrol with a personal trainer, you may be offered a series of baseline health and fitness tests before you start. Some sports-footwear specialists provide gait assessments, too.

Medical checks

Medical testing takes many forms, from blood samples that check how your organs are working to scans that take two- or three-dimensional images of the body, and viewing tests that allow doctors to examine an organ internally. They may be used to assess symptoms or to monitor long-term problems.

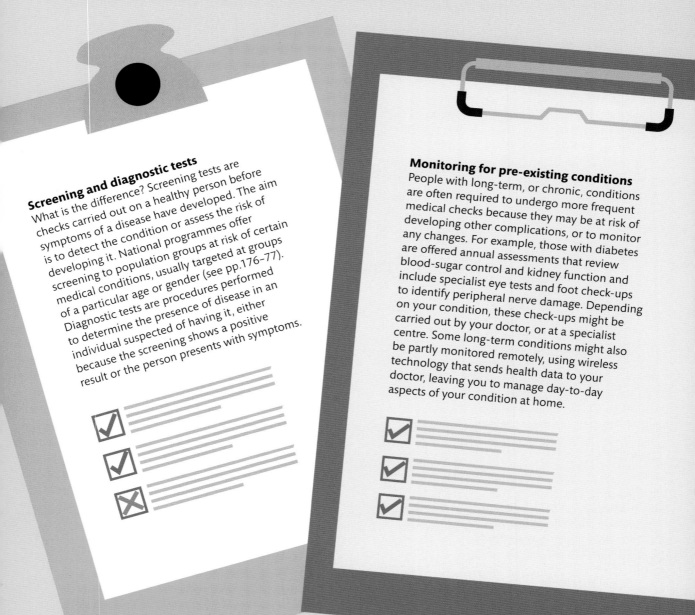

Screening and diagnostic tests

What is the difference? Screening tests are checks carried out on a healthy person before symptoms of a disease have developed. The aim is to detect the condition or assess the risk of developing it. National programmes offer screening to population groups at risk of certain medical conditions, usually targeted at groups of a particular age or gender (see pp.176–77). Diagnostic tests are procedures performed to determine the presence of disease in an individual suspected of having it, either because the screening shows a positive result or the person presents with symptoms.

Monitoring for pre-existing conditions

People with long-term, or chronic, conditions are often required to undergo more frequent medical checks because they may be at risk of developing other complications, or to monitor any changes. For example, those with diabetes are offered annual assessments that review blood-sugar control and kidney function and include specialist eye tests and foot check-ups to identify peripheral nerve damage. Depending on your condition, these check-ups might be carried out by your doctor, or at a specialist centre. Some long-term conditions might also be partly monitored remotely, using wireless technology that sends health data to your doctor, leaving you to manage day-to-day aspects of your condition at home.

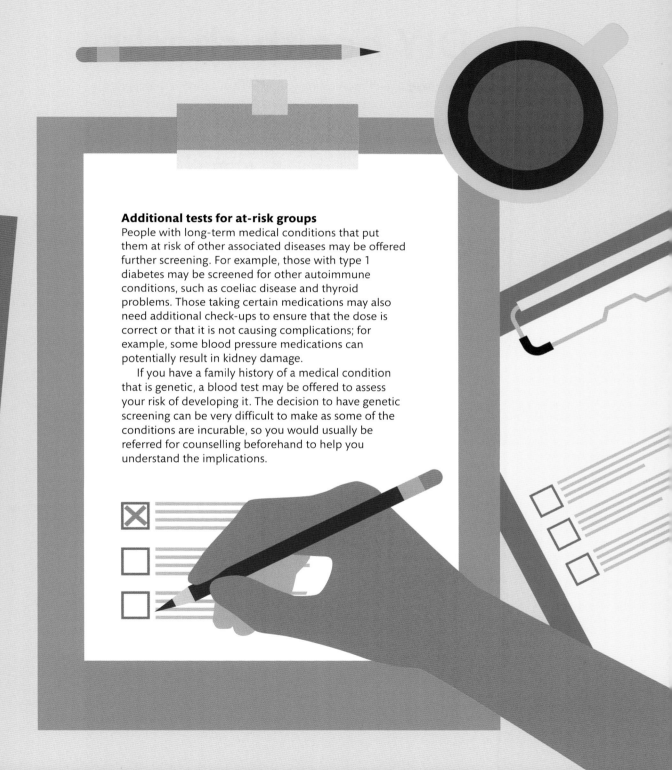

Additional tests for at-risk groups

People with long-term medical conditions that put them at risk of other associated diseases may be offered further screening. For example, those with type 1 diabetes may be screened for other autoimmune conditions, such as coeliac disease and thyroid problems. Those taking certain medications may also need additional check-ups to ensure that the dose is correct or that it is not causing complications; for example, some blood pressure medications can potentially result in kidney damage.

If you have a family history of a medical condition that is genetic, a blood test may be offered to assess your risk of developing it. The decision to have genetic screening can be very difficult to make as some of the conditions are incurable, so you would usually be referred for counselling beforehand to help you understand the implications.

DIY health checks

The advantage of monitoring your health at home is that it gives you a realistic overview of your wellbeing and of any factors that affect it. Keep a diary of all your findings and talk to your doctor if the results appear unusual.

60

Personal checks
You are the person best placed to notice any changes in your health, however subtle. If you have a long-term condition such as diabetes, you will need to check your own blood sugar daily; if you have asthma, you may need to measure your peak airflow. However, it is also important to be aware of common signs and symptoms of other potentially serious health conditions. Set aside time, ideally once a month, to check your body: for example, for lumps or moles (see pp.98–99). Seek medical advice, too, if you notice changes such as blood in your stool or unexplained bloating, abdominal pain, or weight loss.

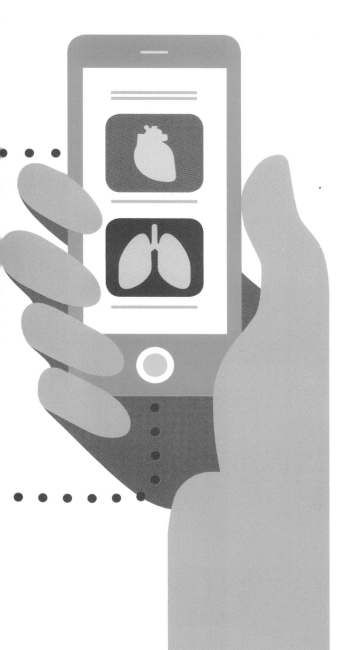

Commercial and online testing

A number of websites enable you to screen yourself for health issues, such as vision problems, and you can use online questionnaires to check for signs of dementia or depression. While these can all be useful indicators, they are not a substitute for medical advice, so you should speak to a health professional, too – taking your results with you.

You can also buy medical testing kits for use at home – online or at your pharmacy – that claim to analyse anything from cholesterol or fertility levels to bowel cancer. Remember, however, that not all companies are quality-assured, so results may not be accurate, and need to be interpreted correctly. Moreover, your doctor can request testing if you present with the relevant symptoms.

Wearable fitness devices

Technological advances have provided many platforms for monitoring your day-to-day health. Wearable gadgets, often linked to phone applications, enable you to track fitness and activity levels, food and calorie intake, even sleep quality. Some have a built-in electrocardiogram (ECG) that monitors heartbeat and rhythm, and there are applications that check oxygen saturation, women's health and fertility, cancerous changes in the skin, and much more. While these devices can be empowering, some applications are more accurate than others, so can give a false-positive or false-negative result. Do not rely solely on this technology; talk to your doctor if you are concerned.

HOME MONITORING EQUIPMENT

There are a number of devices that enable you to monitor your health. Make sure you know how to interpret the results.

- Weighing scales range from simple mechanical devices to sophisticated digital gadgets that can measure body fat, body-water percentage, or muscle mass – a few have built-in Wi-Fi so you can upload data to your phone or tablet.
- A tape measure is useful for measuring your waist (see p.24).
- Home blood pressure monitors allow you to take daily readings. Choose one that measures the pressure in the upper arm and make sure the cuff is the right size for your arm. Have it serviced regularly – at least every two years.
- A blood-oxygen saturation probe gives a digital readout when clipped onto your index finger.
- Blood glucose monitors are essential for anyone with diabetes. Choose one that keeps a record of your results. Some alert you to high or low glucose patterns and even check for ketones, a complication of type 1 diabetes.
- Peak-flow meters test the strength of your exhaled breaths.

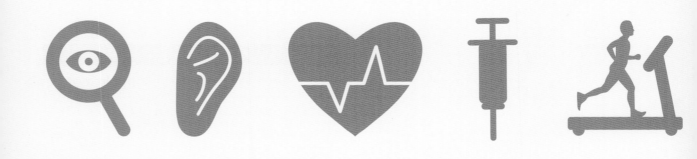

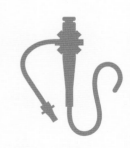

General adult tests

Body weight

It is important to keep to a healthy body weight, as being overweight or underweight can increase your risk of certain disorders. Your doctor may monitor your weight by weighing you and measuring your body mass index (BMI) and waist size.

Weight and health

Your weight depends on your sex, age, height, shape, bone and muscle structure, and fat distribution. It is also influenced by your metabolism (how your body turns food into energy) and lifestyle. Being overweight might not immediately cause health issues, but excess fat can put a strain on your joints and can raise your risk of sleep disorders, heart disease, high blood pressure, and diabetes. It is also important not to be underweight, as this can increase your risk of disorders such as osteoporosis.

Waist and hip size

The doctor may measure your waist to see if you have excess fat around your middle, which can increase your risk of developing diabetes or heart and circulation diseases. The doctor may also measure around the hips and work out your waist–hip ratio, to assess body fat distribution.

Measuring your hips and waist
Use a cloth measuring tape or a piece of string. Wrap the tape around you so it is level and lies flat without digging in.

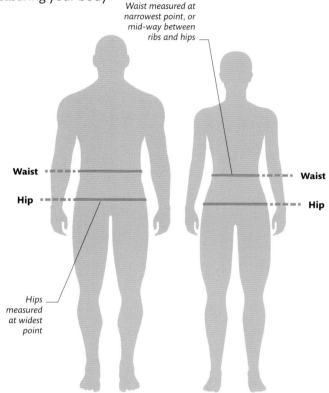

Waist measured at narrowest point, or mid-way between ribs and hips

Waist

Hip

Hips measured at widest point

Waist

Hip

WAIST AND HIP MEASUREMENTS

Weight around the middle usually means that there is more fat near the internal organs, which might influence the way they function.

Formula for waist–hip ratio:

$$\frac{\text{Waist measurement (cm or in)}}{\text{Hip measurement (cm or in)}}$$

Measurements	Gender	Healthy	Moderate risk	High risk
Waist size	Men	<94 cm (37 in)	94–102 cm (37–40 in)	>102 cm (40 in)
	Women	<80 cm (31.5 in)	80–88 cm (31.5–34 in)	>88 cm (34 in)
Waist-hip ratio	Men	<0.9	0.9-0.99	≥1.0
	Women	<0.8	0.8-0.89	≥0.9

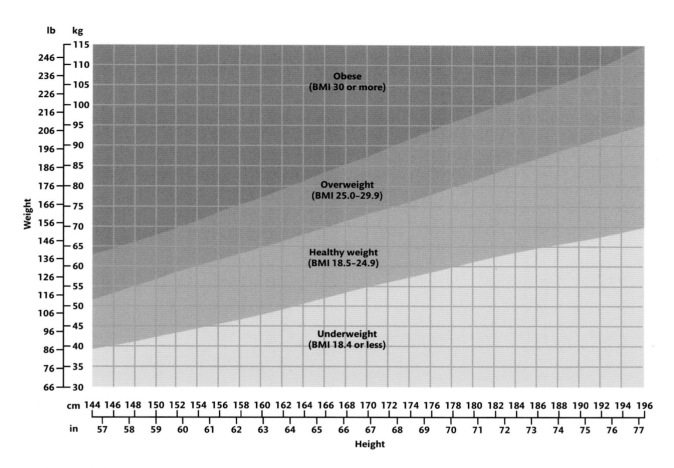

Obese
(BMI 30 or more)

Overweight
(BMI 25.0–29.9)

Healthy weight
(BMI 18.5–24.9)

Underweight
(BMI 18.4 or less)

Weight

Height

Body mass index

Body mass index (BMI) is a calculation based on weight and height. It will show generally whether you are carrying too much or too little weight for someone of your height. It is not a totally accurate guide; for example, some muscular athletes may have a BMI suggesting that they are overweight, and BMI does not indicate fat distribution. In addition, BMI does not distinguish between men and women. However, it is still a quick and useful tool to help you assess weight-related health risks.

Adult BMI chart

You can check whether you fall in a healthy weight range by using the weight/height chart above, or by calculating it yourself (see below, left). This chart shows the ranges for adults only.

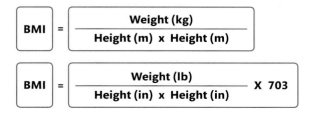

$$BMI = \frac{Weight\ (kg)}{Height\ (m)\ x\ Height\ (m)}$$

$$BMI = \frac{Weight\ (lb)}{Height\ (in)\ x\ Height\ (in)}\ X\ 703$$

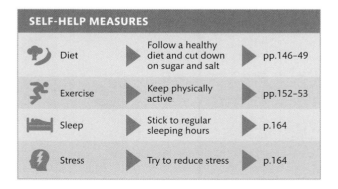

SELF-HELP MEASURES

	Diet		Follow a healthy diet and cut down on sugar and salt	pp.146–49
	Exercise		Keep physically active	pp.152–53
	Sleep		Stick to regular sleeping hours	p.164
	Stress		Try to reduce stress	p.164

Your heart and circulation

Your heart and blood vessels – arteries, veins, and capillaries – form the transport network that carries blood to every cell in your body, supplying the cells with oxygen, nutrients, and other vital chemicals, and removing wastes. The heart beats continually to pump blood through the blood vessels; muscles and valves in the blood vessels also keep the blood moving freely.

Structure of the heart
The heart is divided vertically into two halves. Each half consists of an upper chamber (atrium) that receives blood from the veins, and a lower chamber (ventricle) that pumps blood into the arteries. One-way valves prevent backflow of blood.

Pumping blood
Located in the chest behind the breastbone, the heart is a fist-sized, hollow, muscular organ that pumps about 60–70 times a minute (when you are at rest) to ensure a continual flow of fresh blood to all parts of the body. Its right-hand chambers receive oxygen-depleted blood from the body and pump it to the lungs to be oxygenated. The oxygenated blood returns to the left-hand chambers, where it is pumped around the body, eventually returning to the right side of the heart to repeat the cycle.

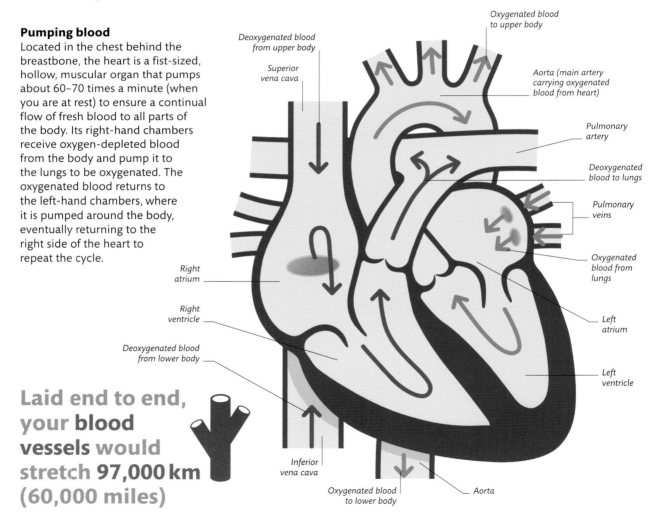

Deoxygenated blood from upper body

Superior vena cava

Oxygenated blood to upper body

Aorta (main artery carrying oxygenated blood from heart)

Pulmonary artery

Deoxygenated blood to lungs

Pulmonary veins

Oxygenated blood from lungs

Right atrium

Right ventricle

Deoxygenated blood from lower body

Left atrium

Left ventricle

Inferior vena cava

Oxygenated blood to lower body

Aorta

Laid end to end, your blood vessels would stretch 97,000 km (60,000 miles)

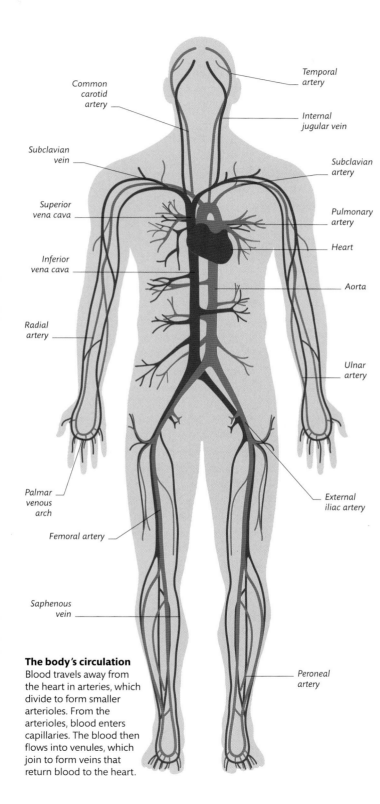

Common carotid artery

Temporal artery

Internal jugular vein

Subclavian vein

Subclavian artery

Superior vena cava

Pulmonary artery

Heart

Inferior vena cava

Aorta

Radial artery

Ulnar artery

Palmar venous arch

External iliac artery

Femoral artery

Saphenous vein

Peroneal artery

The body's circulation
Blood travels away from the heart in arteries, which divide to form smaller arterioles. From the arterioles, blood enters capillaries. The blood then flows into venules, which join to form veins that return blood to the heart.

CHECKING THE HEART AND CIRCULATION

Problems with your heart and circulation are potentially serious, as they could lead to conditions such as a heart attack or a stroke. Basic checks of cardiovascular health include measuring your blood pressure and your heart rate and rhythm. More sophisticated checks include electrocardiography (ECG) and ultrasound imaging such as echocardiography and scanning for an aortic aneurysm.

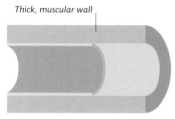

Thick, muscular wall

Structure of an artery
Arteries have thick, muscular walls to withstand the high pressure of blood pumped from the heart. Arteries can dilate or constrict to help regulate blood pressure.

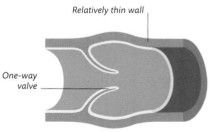

Relatively thin wall

One-way valve

Structure of a vein
Veins have relatively thin, stretchy walls so that they can cope with any increases in blood flow. Large veins contain one-way valves to prevent backflow of blood.

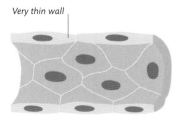

Very thin wall

Structure of a capillary
Capillaries are the smallest blood vessels. They have walls only one cell thick to allow oxygen, nutrients, and wastes to pass into and out of the blood easily.

Measuring blood pressure

The pressure of blood in your arteries as your heart beats can reveal how well your heart and blood vessels are working and show any signs of high blood pressure, or hypertension. Hypertension over a sustained period can lead to potentially serious health problems.

Systole
The ventricles contract, forcing blood into the pulmonary arteries and aorta. The blood pulses at high pressure through these blood vessels to the lungs and body tissues, respectively.

The **heart pumps** about **6 litres** (10½ pints) around the body once every minute

Diastole
The heart muscle relaxes and the atria fill with blood from the veins. The blood then passes from the atria into the ventricles. Blood is not being pumped out of the heart so blood pressure is lower.

What happens when the heart beats
Each time the heart beats, the arteries pulse with blood so the pressure inside them rises and falls in waves. Each heartbeat is triggered by a signal from the heart's natural pacemaker. When the ventricles (lower chambers) contract – systole – blood is forced out of the heart. This is followed by diastole, when the heart muscle relaxes ready for the next beat.

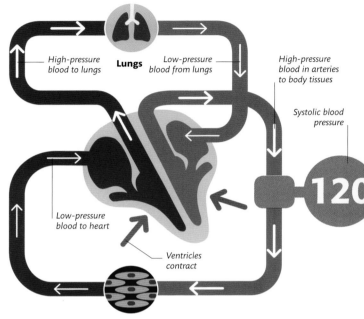

High-pressure blood to lungs
Lungs
Low-pressure blood from lungs
High-pressure blood in arteries to body tissues
Systolic blood pressure
Low-pressure blood to heart
Ventricles contract
120
Body tissues

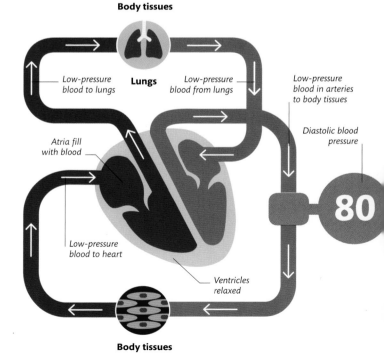

Low-pressure blood to lungs
Lungs
Low-pressure blood from lungs
Low-pressure blood in arteries to body tissues
Diastolic blood pressure
Atria fill with blood
Low-pressure blood to heart
Ventricles relaxed
80
Body tissues

Blood pressure measurement

Blood pressure is measured with a device called a sphygmomanometer, consisting of an inflatable cuff and a monitor. The doctor fits the cuff around your upper arm. The cuff is connected with a tube to a pump to inflate it, and to a digital monitor to measure the blood pressure and display the reading. When you are sitting comfortably, with your forearm resting on a flat surface, air is pumped into the cuff. You may feel a slightly uncomfortable squeezing. The air is then slowly released, and the monitor automatically measures the maximum (systolic) and minimum (diastolic) pressure.

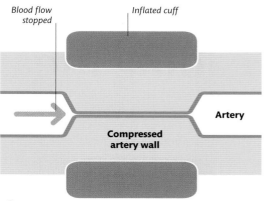

Blood flow stopped

Inflated cuff

Artery

Compressed artery wall

❶ The cuff is inflated

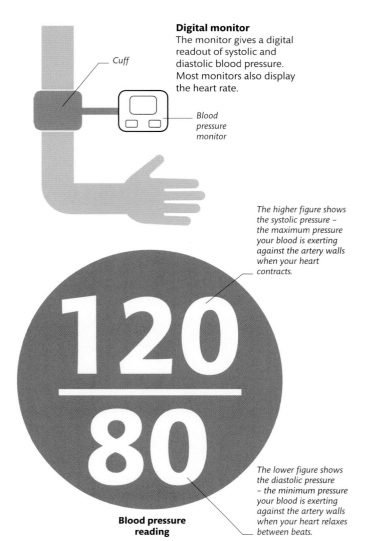

Digital monitor
The monitor gives a digital readout of systolic and diastolic blood pressure. Most monitors also display the heart rate.

Cuff

Blood pressure monitor

The higher figure shows the systolic pressure – the maximum pressure your blood is exerting against the artery walls when your heart contracts.

120
―――
80

The lower figure shows the diastolic pressure – the minimum pressure your blood is exerting against the artery walls when your heart relaxes between beats.

Blood pressure reading

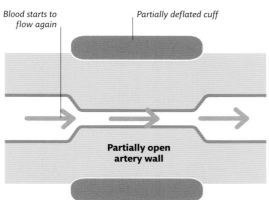

Blood starts to flow again

Partially deflated cuff

Partially open artery wall

❷ Systolic pressure measured

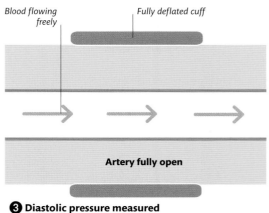

Blood flowing freely

Fully deflated cuff

Artery fully open

❸ Diastolic pressure measured

What your blood pressure reading means

High blood pressure – also known as hypertension – is a long-term medical condition that can lead to cardiovascular disease. However, this "silent killer" is both preventable and treatable. Along with other lifestyle choices, what we eat and drink can have a direct effect on our blood pressure.

Blood pressure at rest
Your blood pressure may go up when you exercise or rush around. It then settles when you are at rest and this is when you should measure it.

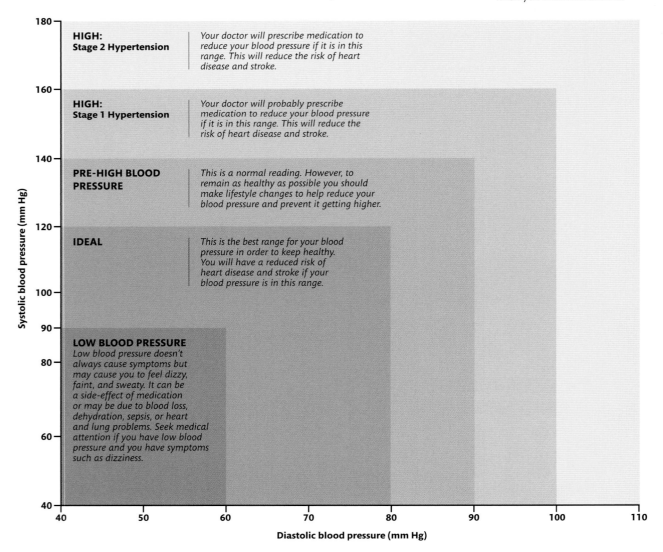

Systolic blood pressure (mm Hg)

HIGH:
Stage 2 Hypertension
Your doctor will prescribe medication to reduce your blood pressure if it is in this range. This will reduce the risk of heart disease and stroke.

HIGH:
Stage 1 Hypertension
Your doctor will probably prescribe medication to reduce your blood pressure if it is in this range. This will reduce the risk of heart disease and stroke.

PRE-HIGH BLOOD PRESSURE
This is a normal reading. However, to remain as healthy as possible you should make lifestyle changes to help reduce your blood pressure and prevent it getting higher.

IDEAL
This is the best range for your blood pressure in order to keep healthy. You will have a reduced risk of heart disease and stroke if your blood pressure is in this range.

LOW BLOOD PRESSURE
Low blood pressure doesn't always cause symptoms but may cause you to feel dizzy, faint, and sweaty. It can be a side-effect of medication or may be due to blood loss, dehydration, sepsis, or heart and lung problems. Seek medical attention if you have low blood pressure and you have symptoms such as dizziness.

Diastolic blood pressure (mm Hg)

Interpreting your results

Your blood pressure is written as two numbers, such as 140/90 (see pp.28–29). When only one of these figures is high and the other one is normal, you should use the high one to determine which blood pressure category (see opposite) you are in. You should not usually rely on one reading alone to decide if your blood pressure is raised as things such as stress and anxiety can temporarily make your blood pressure go up. Usually you should monitor it twice a day for at least a week. You should see your doctor if your home readings (see panel, right) are above 135/85.

Why is high blood pressure dangerous?

Although there are rarely any symptoms of high blood pressure, if it is left untreated the heart gradually becomes enlarged and less efficient. Slowly, the blood vessels, kidneys, eyes, and other parts of the body can become damaged. As blood pressure goes up, artery walls become thicker and stronger and arteries become narrower, threatening to slow or even stop blood flow. This increases the risk of heart attack.

SELF-MONITORING

Taking your own blood pressure using a home monitor has become very popular. You can purchase reliable machines from shops or online. Home blood pressure machines usually have a standard upper arm cuff, but there are wrist cuff monitors available, though they may give a slightly higher and less accurate reading. Home monitors are not suitable if you have an irregular pulse.

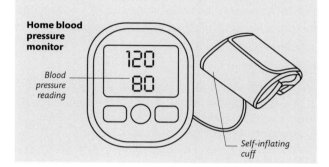

Home blood pressure monitor

Blood pressure reading

Self-inflating cuff

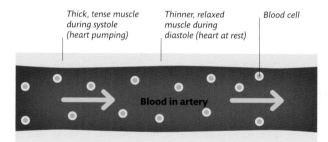

Thick, tense muscle during systole (heart pumping)

Thinner, relaxed muscle during diastole (heart at rest)

Blood cell

Blood in artery

NORMAL BLOOD PRESSURE

Healthy arteries
A normal blood pressure changes from a high, as the heart pumps, to a low, when it relaxes. The muscles in our artery walls respond to these fluctuations by tensing and relaxing in rhythm.

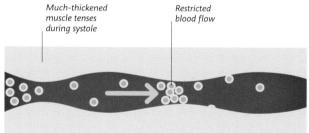

Much-thickened muscle tenses during systole

Restricted blood flow

CHRONIC HIGH BLOOD PRESSURE

Narrowing arteries
If your blood pressure is high, your arteries have to work harder to resist the pressure, so their walls become stronger and thicker. As your arteries get narrower, blood pressure rises further.

Worldwide, the **number of people** with **uncontrolled hypertension** is estimated to **exceed 1 billion**

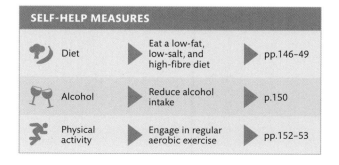

SELF-HELP MEASURES

Diet	Eat a low-fat, low-salt, and high-fibre diet	pp.146–49
Alcohol	Reduce alcohol intake	p.150
Physical activity	Engage in regular aerobic exercise	pp.152–53

Checking your heart rate

Your heart rate – also known as your pulse rate – is the number of times your heart beats per minute. The rate varies from person to person, and also according to a wide range of other factors, such as level of activity, stress, emotion, age, and substances such as caffeine.

SELF-MONITORING

Personal fitness monitors allow you to automatically keep track of your heart rate at any time. They record your heart rate at rest as well as during exercise and work. They can be used for fitness training but the records can also be sent to your doctor for monitoring of your heart rate.

Although there are considerable variations in heart rate, in general, a lower heart rate at rest implies more efficient heart function and better cardiovascular fitness, with an associated reduced risk of a heart attack.

Measuring the heart rate
Your doctor may measure your heart rate at the same time as measuring your blood pressure with an automatic blood pressure monitor (see pp.28–29).
Your heart rate varies according to how much physical activity you have been doing. To get the most accurate reading, it should be measured after you have been at rest for at least five minutes. This is known as your resting heart rate. To improve the accuracy of the measurements, it is important that the readings are taken before you've taken any stimulants, such as caffeine, or medication. You should also try to ensure that the readings are taken at the same time of day.

You can also measure it yourself (see panel, above), using a personal heart rate monitor, many types of wrist fitness tracker monitors and smart watches, or simply by counting your pulse rate. Your pulse can be felt in your neck or wrist and should be taken using two fingers.

What the results might mean
You can get a more accurate picture if you average out several readings. Although it can be normal for you to have a pulse rate outside the typical range for healthy adults (see below), it would be sensible to see your doctor if this is the case.

Assessing your heart rate
Your heart usually beats in a regular rhythm. An irregular pulse can be caused by a medical problem, anxiety, or be the result of having too much caffeine. If you have an irregular pulse and it persists, you should see a doctor.

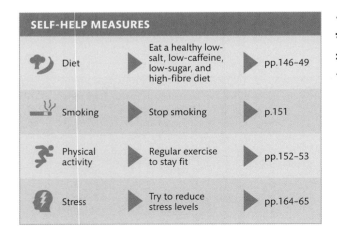

SELF-HELP MEASURES

Diet	Eat a healthy low-salt, low-caffeine, low-sugar, and high-fibre diet	pp.146–49
Smoking	Stop smoking	p.151
Physical activity	Regular exercise to stay fit	pp.152–53
Stress	Try to reduce stress levels	pp.164–65

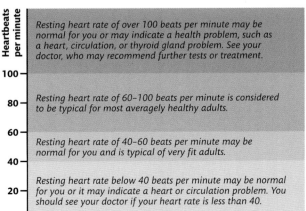

Heartbeats per minute

Resting heart rate of over 100 beats per minute may be normal for you or may indicate a health problem, such as a heart, circulation, or thyroid gland problem. See your doctor, who may recommend further tests or treatment.

100 —

Resting heart rate of 60–100 beats per minute is considered to be typical for most averagely healthy adults.

80 —

60 —

Resting heart rate of 40–60 beats per minute may be normal for you and is typical of very fit adults.

40 —

Resting heart rate below 40 beats per minute may be normal for you or it may indicate a heart or circulation problem. You should see your doctor if your heart rate is less than 40.

20 —

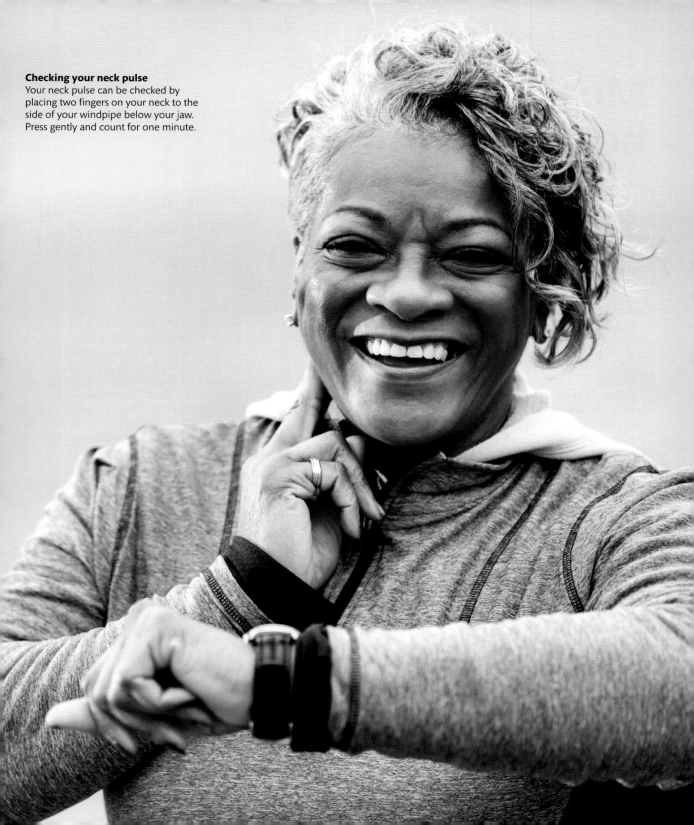

Checking your neck pulse
Your neck pulse can be checked by placing two fingers on your neck to the side of your windpipe below your jaw. Press gently and count for one minute.

Measuring your heart's rhythm

Your heart has a natural electrical circuit that is continually active. This electrical activity starts in the upper right chamber and travels along a conducting pathway to the lower chambers, causing the heart to pump and creating your heartbeat. Although it is not possible to visualize the electrical circuit directly, the electrical pattern can be visualized on an electrocardiogram (ECG).

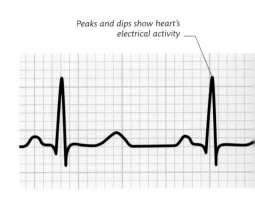

Peaks and dips show heart's electrical activity

What the test involves

An ECG can be used to diagnose a possible cause for symptoms such as chest pain, dizziness, breathlessness, or palpitations. It can also be taken prior to an operation to check the heart's health, as part of an insurance medical, or if there is a family history of heart problems at a young age. For the test you will lie down on an examination couch. The technician will apply six small sticky pads – called electrodes – to the front of your chest and one to each arm and leg. If you are a woman, you may be asked to remove your bra and wear a gown instead. Occasionally men with very hairy chests will be asked to shave a small area so that the pads can stick to the skin. Wires from the ECG machine will then be clipped to each pad. You will be asked to keep still while the recording is made, which only takes about 30 seconds and is completely painless.

What the results mean

The ECG shows how fast your heart is beating (see pp.32–33) and whether your heartbeat is regular. It may indicate that your heart is healthy and beating normally. However, it may reveal features of a heart attack and can also indicate if you have had a heart attack in the past. Other changes on the ECG may indicate abnormalities in the normal electrical conduction pathway or in the heart muscle, as well as an abnormally fast or slow heart rate. Sometimes, you may be sent for further tests such as an ambulatory ECG or an exercise ECG (see pp.36–37).

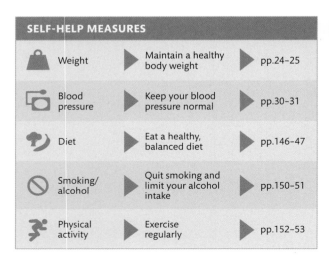

SELF-HELP MEASURES

	Weight	▶	Maintain a healthy body weight	▶	pp.24–25
	Blood pressure	▶	Keep your blood pressure normal	▶	pp.30–31
	Diet	▶	Eat a healthy, balanced diet	▶	pp.146–47
	Smoking/ alcohol	▶	Quit smoking and limit your alcohol intake	▶	pp.150–51
	Physical activity	▶	Exercise regularly	▶	pp.152–53

SELF-MONITORING

It is possible for you to do a mini-ECG recording yourself using some of the latest smart watches or specific hand-held devices. These are linked to an app on your mobile phone. They produce an ECG tracing from a section of your ECG. The tracings are particularly useful if you have palpitations or there are concerns that you have an irregular heartbeat, because an ECG record can then be done at the exact time the symptoms occur and may help to diagnose conditions such as atrial fibrillation.

Graph paper allows exact measurements to be taken

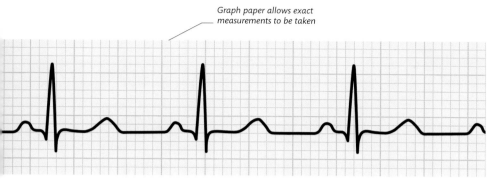

Normal ECG
The ECG is a series of tracings printed onto graph paper that give a graphical representation of the electrical activity of your heart at that particular time. This image shows a tracing from one section of an ECG of a person with a normal heartbeat.

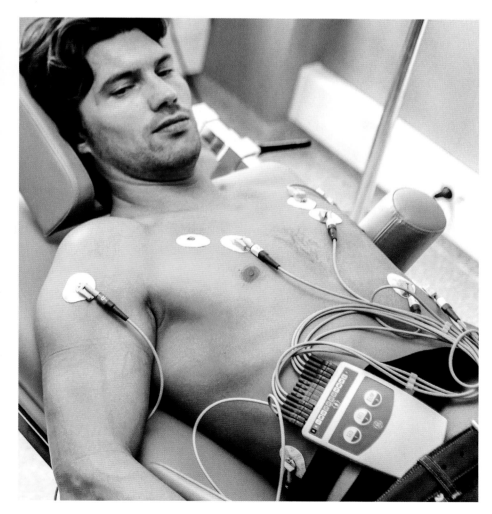

Undergoing an ECG
A resting ECG is taken while you lie comfortably on your back, with the electrodes that take the measurements attached to your skin.

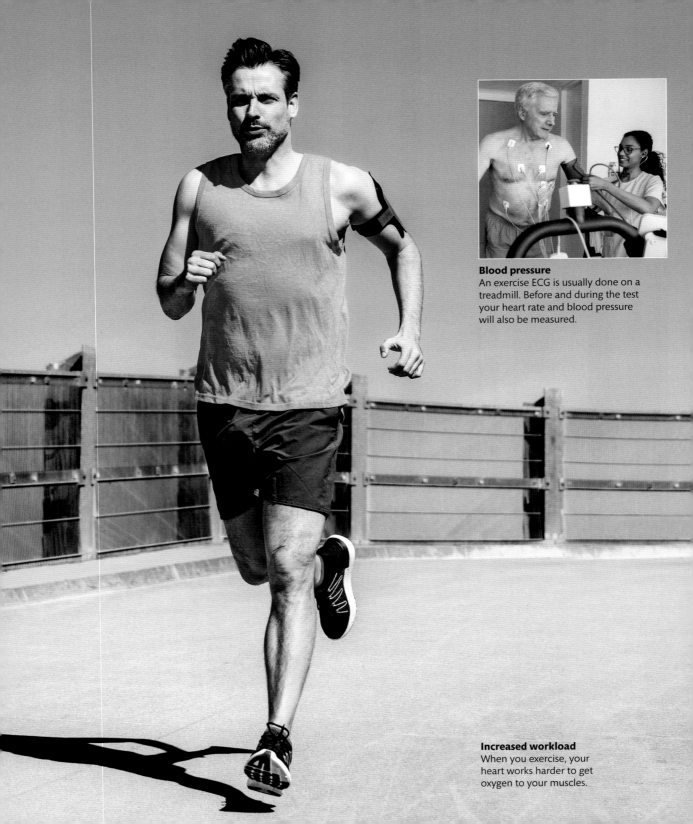

Blood pressure
An exercise ECG is usually done on a treadmill. Before and during the test your heart rate and blood pressure will also be measured.

Increased workload
When you exercise, your heart works harder to get oxygen to your muscles.

Exercise electrocardiogram

An exercise electrocardiogram (ECG) is a graphical recording of the electrical activity of your heart while you exercise. Exercise causes your heart to beat faster and this test can see how your heart copes with the increased workload.

What to expect from the test

This test detects changes in the heart's electrical activity that may only become apparent when your heart speeds up, such as during exercise or when under stress. For this reason, it is also known as a stress test. It can be used to find a cause for symptoms such as breathlessness, chest pain, or palpitations that occur when you exert yourself. Although this test is usually only recommended if your doctor is concerned about your heart, it may occasionally be offered as part of a well-person check by your health insurance company or to assess your fitness for a new exercise regime. It is also used to check your heart after a heart attack or heart procedure.

This test requires you to walk on a moving treadmill that gradually gets faster and steeper over about 10 minutes. Occasionally, you may be asked to pedal a stationary bike instead. You will be connected to an ECG machine via sticky pads on your chest and also have your blood pressure and heart rate monitored. It is not a competition and the test will be stopped if you complain of chest pain, shortness of breath, feel unwell, or if there are certain changes on your ECG tracing. If you are not able to do the exercise required, there are other tests, such as a nuclear scan, which can provide similar information to the exercise ECG.

What the results mean

Your exercise ECG tracing may be normal, which can be very reassuring for you. However, it may also show changes that suggest you may have reduced blood flow to your heart muscle. This can be due to narrowing in the arteries supplying your heart. In this case, your doctor will recommend that you have further tests to look at these blood vessels in more detail.

Reaching your target heart rate
During an exercise ECG, the intensity of the activity will increase until you reach a target heart rate set by your doctor. This may be 85 per cent of your maximum heart rate. Once you've reached your target heart rate, the intensity is gradually decreased so that you cool down, rather than stopping abruptly.

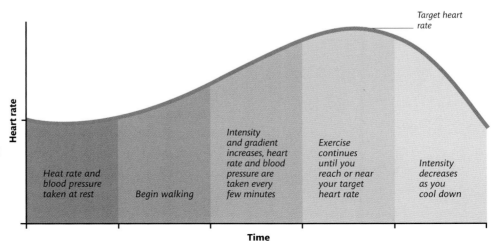

Target heart rate

Heart rate

Heat rate and blood pressure taken at rest

Begin walking

Intensity and gradient increases, heart rate and blood pressure are taken every few minutes

Exercise continues until you reach or near your target heart rate

Intensity decreases as you cool down

Time

Echocardiography

An echocardiogram is a heart scan that uses sound waves to create images of your heart on a screen. This is an excellent way for your doctor to also assess the size of your heart, how efficiently it is pumping, and whether the valves are leaking or have thickened.

Heart scan
A technician places a probe on the chest of a person having an echocardiogram and Doppler scan. The additional electrodes, attached to his chest, measure his heartbeat.

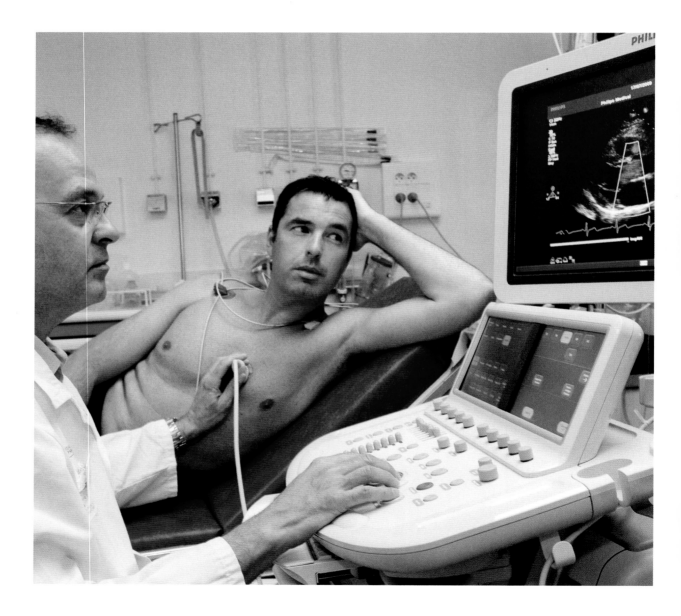

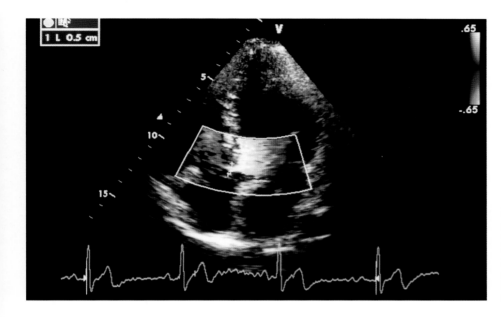

Doppler scan
An echocardiogram shows the four chambers of the heart, while the blue and red colours are the result of the Doppler ultrasound scan. This shows the flow of blood through the heart.

What the test involves

You may be sent for an echocardiogram if you complain of breathlessness or chest pain or have been found to have a heart murmur or high blood pressure. You may also have one after a heart attack to see if your heart muscle is damaged.

The most common type of echo is called a transthoracic scan. A small probe, which transmits sound waves, will be placed on various areas of your chest wall. It is painless, but you may feel some pressure. You will be asked to remove your top clothes and will be given a gown to wear if necessary. The echo is performed while you are lying on a bed on your left side. The room lights will be dimmed so that the screen can be easily seen.

The virtual moving picture of the inside of your heart will show the heart's general structure, the valves opening and closing, and the heart muscle moving. At the same time, a Doppler scan is done, which shows the speed and direction of blood flowing through your heart.

What the results might mean

The echo may show your heart is normal, which is very reassuring. It may also help to diagnose heart failure, valve problems, and heart muscle disorders. If the echo indicates a heart problem, you may be prescribed medication or be referred for further tests, which may lead to heart surgery.

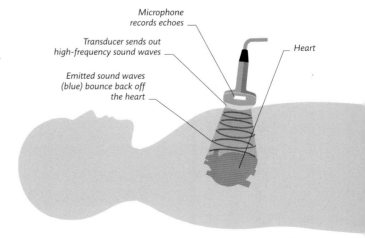

Microphone records echoes

Transducer sends out high-frequency sound waves

Heart

Emitted sound waves (blue) bounce back off the heart

Sonic picture

An ultrasound scan is made with high-frequency sound waves. The sound waves bounce off solid substances, such as organs or bone, and the returning echoes are processed by a computer to generate an image.

Abdominal aortic aneurysm scan

The aorta is the main blood vessel that carries oxygen-rich blood from your heart to the rest of your body. As you get older, the wall of your aorta can weaken and swell. This bulge is called an aneurysm. It is more common in the part of the aorta situated in the abdomen.

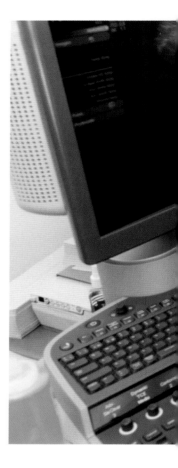

What the test involves
You are more likely to have an aneurysm if you are male and you smoke, and have high blood pressure or high cholesterol. Sometimes there may be a history of an aneurysm in a close relative. You may be unaware that you have an aneurysm as it rarely causes symptoms until it ruptures. A ruptured aneurysm is a medical emergency as it causes severe internal bleeding and is often fatal, so early detection can be life-saving. You may be offered a scan if you are at increased risk – for example, if you are a man over age 65.

The ultrasound scan will involve you lying on a bed with your top clothes pulled up. Some gel will be put on your abdomen and a probe that transmits the sound waves is placed on it. Images of your aorta will appear on a screen and the width of it will be measured to check for an aneurysm.

What the results might mean
You will usually be given your results straight away. It is very reassuring if your scan shows that your aorta is normal and you will not need further scans. However, if a small aneurysm is found then you will be called back for regular repeat scans, as aneurysms usually get larger over time. If an aneurysm reaches 5.5cm (2³⁄₁₆ in) then it is more likely that you will be considered for surgery as the risk of rupture is significant once it is larger than this.

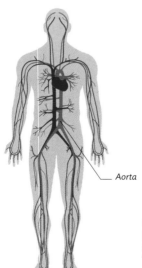

Aorta

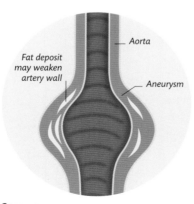

Fat deposit may weaken artery wall

Aorta

Aneurysm

Common aneurysm
Blood pressure in the aorta can cause a weakened area of the artery wall to bulge. The bulge will continue to grow and has the potential to burst, which is often fatal.

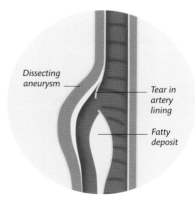

Dissecting aneurysm

Tear in artery lining

Fatty deposit

Dissecting aneurysm
A dissecting aneurysm occurs when there is a tear in the inner wall of the artery. Blood seeps into the artery wall, causing it to swell and the wall to thin. This is a medical emergency.

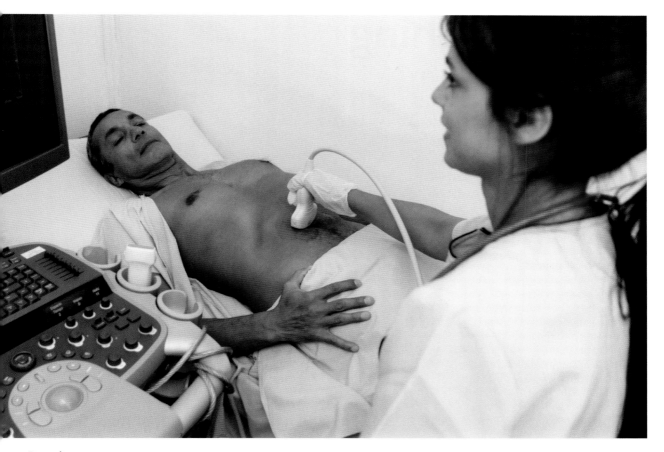

Detecting an aneurysm
A technician will use a probe, called a transducer, to bounce sound waves off your aorta. This echo information is then used to create an image of the aorta on a computer screen.

TABLE OF RESULTS

Diameter of aorta	What this means
Less than 3cm (1³⁄₁₆ in) across	This is normal and no aneurysm is detected
3–4.4cm across (1³⁄₁₆–1¾ in)	Small aneurysm; manage size through lifestyle changes
4.5–5.4cm across (1⅞–2⅛ in)	Medium aneurysm; manage size through lifestyle changes
Over 5.5cm (2³⁄₁₆ in) across	Large aneurysm; likely to require surgery to prevent rupture

SELF-HELP MEASURES

Blood pressure	Maintain a normal blood pressure	pp.30–31
Diet	Cut out saturated fat from your diet	pp.146–49
Smoking	Stop smoking	p.151
Exercise	Keep physically active	pp.152–53

How breathing works

Breathing is the process by which the body takes in oxygen, which cells use to generate energy from food. There are two main elements: ventilation – the movements of the chest (inhalation and exhalation), and gas exchange – the transfer of oxygen and carbon dioxide inside your lungs.

The breathing process

The action of breathing muscles draws air in through the nose, mouth, or both. The air passes down the trachea (windpipe) into the two bronchi (the main airways into the lungs). From here, it passes through smaller airways until it reaches tiny pouches called alveoli. Here, oxygen passes into the bloodstream, which carries it to the heart and then to the body tissues. Blood that has released its oxygen is returned via the heart to the lungs. This low-oxygen blood also releases waste carbon dioxide into the alveoli, from where it is exhaled.

An adult breathes at least 7.5 litres (13 pints) of air per minute

The lungs

The lungs are contained in a slippery, double-layered membrane called the pleural membrane, which allows the lungs to expand freely inside the chest as they are moved by the breathing muscles, principally the diaphragm.

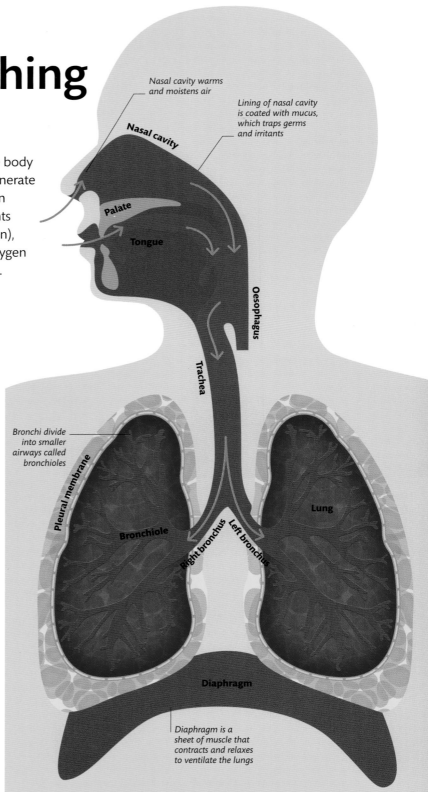

Nasal cavity warms and moistens air

Lining of nasal cavity is coated with mucus, which traps germs and irritants

Nasal cavity

Palate

Tongue

Oesophagus

Trachea

Bronchi divide into smaller airways called bronchioles

Pleural membrane

Bronchiole

Right bronchus

Left bronchus

Lung

Diaphragm

Diaphragm is a sheet of muscle that contracts and relaxes to ventilate the lungs

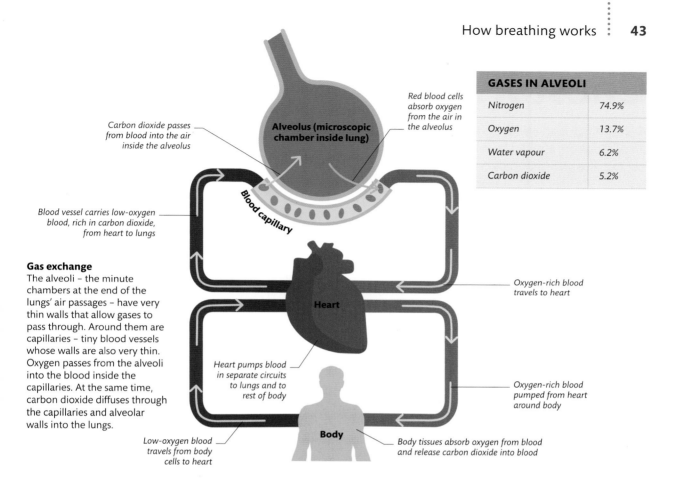

Carbon dioxide passes from blood into the air inside the alveolus

Alveolus (microscopic chamber inside lung)

Red blood cells absorb oxygen from the air in the alveolus

Blood capillary

Blood vessel carries low-oxygen blood, rich in carbon dioxide, from heart to lungs

Heart

Oxygen-rich blood travels to heart

Heart pumps blood in separate circuits to lungs and to rest of body

Oxygen-rich blood pumped from heart around body

Body

Low-oxygen blood travels from body cells to heart

Body tissues absorb oxygen from blood and release carbon dioxide into blood

GASES IN ALVEOLI	
Nitrogen	74.9%
Oxygen	13.7%
Water vapour	6.2%
Carbon dioxide	5.2%

Gas exchange

The alveoli – the minute chambers at the end of the lungs' air passages – have very thin walls that allow gases to pass through. Around them are capillaries – tiny blood vessels whose walls are also very thin. Oxygen passes from the alveoli into the blood inside the capillaries. At the same time, carbon dioxide diffuses through the capillaries and alveolar walls into the lungs.

LUNG FUNCTION TESTS

Tests are used to assess how well your lungs and airways are getting oxygen into your body. Chest X-rays (see p.44) show the structures inside your lungs, to reveal any problems such as fluid or air around your lungs. Peak flow tests (see p.45) and spirometry (see pp.46–47) measure how effectively you can breathe in and out, and lung volume tests (see pp.48–49) show how much air your lungs can hold. Pulse oximetry (see p.51) and exercise capacity testing (see p.50) show how much oxygen is reaching your body tissues.

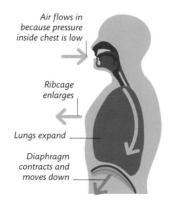

Air flows in because pressure inside chest is low

Ribcage enlarges

Lungs expand

Diaphragm contracts and moves down

Inhalation

When the diaphragm contracts, it flattens and moves down while muscles between the ribs contract to pull the ribs outwards. As the chest and lungs expand, they draw air in through the airways.

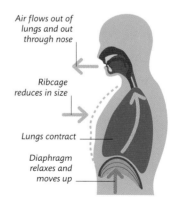

Air flows out of lungs and out through nose

Ribcage reduces in size

Lungs contract

Diaphragm relaxes and moves up

Exhalation

The rib muscles relax and the diaphragm becomes more domed as it too relaxes, causing the chest and lungs to contract in size. Air in the lungs is pushed out of the body via the airways.

Chest X-ray

A chest X-ray is an image of your chest taken using a small amount of X-ray radiation. It might be ordered by your doctor to check your lungs but can also give information about your heart size, ribs, and other bones. It is a very quick test and easy to do.

What the test involves

Once you have arrived at the clinic or hospital, if you are female, you will be asked if you could be pregnant, since the X-rays could harm a developing baby. If you are not a pregnant woman, you will be taken to a changing cubicle to remove your upper clothing (including an underwired bra or neck jewellery) and to put on a gown. In the X-ray room the radiographer will ask you to stand against the machine and take a breath in. The X-ray picture is taken, but you won't feel anything. The X-ray will be sent to your doctor to explain to you.

A healthy chest X-ray

X-rays pass through less dense tissues, such as lungs, and darken the X-ray-detecting plate. Harder tissues, such as bone and cartilage, absorb X-rays. The darkness in this image indicates the lungs are full of air and healthy. Only the largest air passages, near the heart in the centre, are pale, since they are hardened with cartilage.

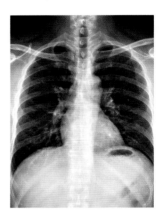

Having a chest X-ray

Healthcare professionals position the patient against a screen containing an X-ray-detecting plate. The X-ray generator (out of shot) then shines a beam of X-rays through the patient's tissues, creating an image on the plate.

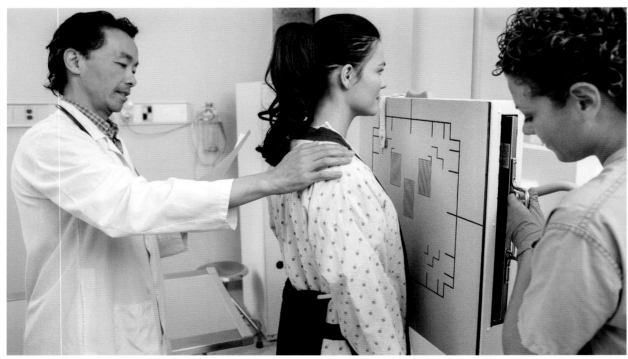

Measuring peak flow

Peak flow, or peak expiratory flow (PEF), is a measurement of the maximum rate at which you can blow air out from your lungs. It is done with a handheld device called a peak flow meter. Your doctor or nurse may ask you to do a peak flow test in order to diagnose or monitor asthma.

What the test involves
The peak flow meter is a hollow device with a scale on the side and a disposable mouthpiece for hygiene. The doctor will ask you to blow as hard as you can into the mouthpiece. This is done three times, and the highest reading is compared to a chart of expected measurements (below) for someone your age, sex, and height. If it is much lower than expected, you might have narrowed airways, and you may be referred for spirometry (see pp.46–47). If asthma is confirmed, sometimes you are given a peak flow meter to monitor your readings at home, to help you recognize when your asthma is not well controlled.

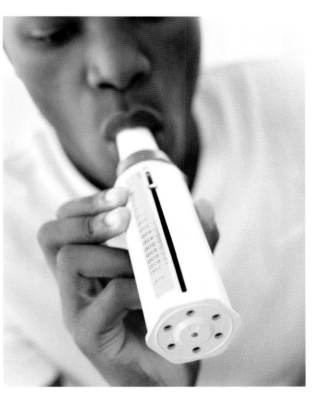

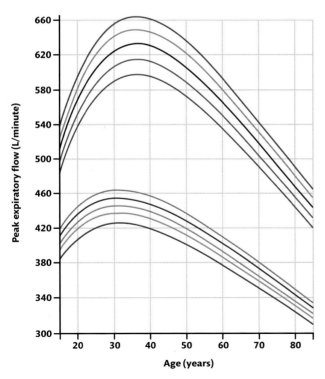

KEY

Men's height
- 190 cm / 75 in
- 183 cm / 72 in
- 175 cm / 69 in
- 167 cm / 66 in
- 160 cm / 63 in

Women's height
- 183 cm / 72 in
- 175 cm / 69 in
- 167 cm / 66 in
- 160 cm / 63 in
- 152 cm / 60 in

Using a peak flow meter
You take a deep breath in. Making sure your lips form a secure seal around the mouthpiece, you then blow into the device as hard as possible.

Predicted values
This graph of "normal" peak flow values was drawn from data from white populations. In estimating your predicted value, your doctor might use values specific to your ethnicity or country. If using a peak flow meter longterm, you might have your own expected values based on your personal best.

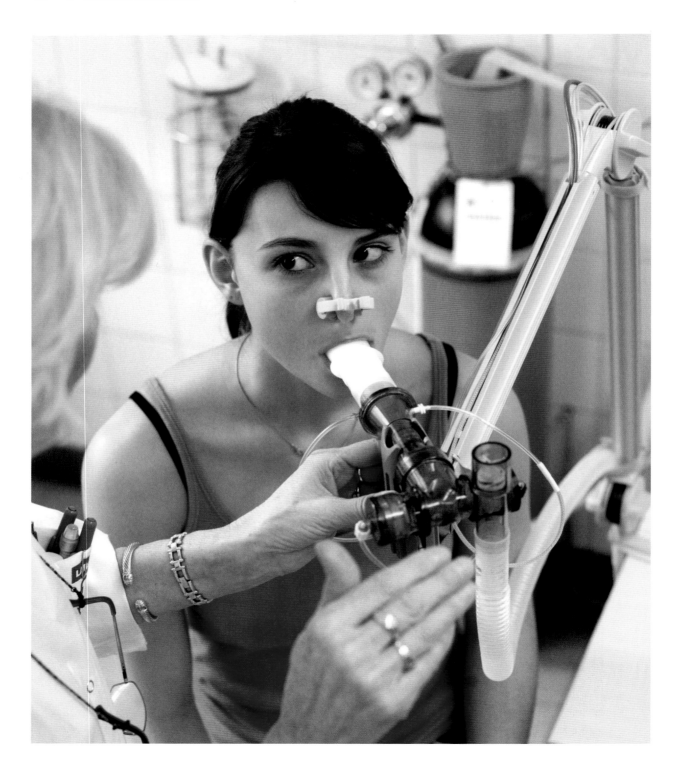

Spirometry

Spirometry looks at how fast and how much you can exhale in one breath. It takes two key measurements – the volume of air you can exhale, or "expire", in the first second of breathing out, and the total volume you can expire. This test can reveal lung problems before symptoms develop.

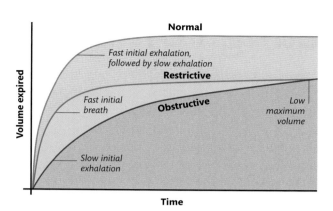

Volume curve
Someone with normal lungs breathes out quickly in the first second, then exhalation slows. Someone with a restrictive problem follows the same pattern, but reaches a lower maximum volume. Someone with an obstructive disorder also has a low maximum volume, but breathes out slowly and takes longer to reach that maximum.

What the test involves

Spirometry can be used to monitor illnesses and assess your health before an operation. It is also used to diagnose the cause of respiratory problems, such as cough or breathing difficulty, including chronic obstructive pulmonary disease (COPD). If you smoke, you may be advised to stop 24 hours before the test. You may also need to avoid alcohol, exercise, or having a heavy meal a few hours beforehand. If you are on inhaled medication, you may be asked to stop using it before the test. In addition, wear loose clothing that will allow you to breathe freely.

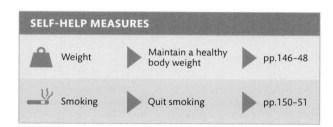

SELF-HELP MEASURES

Weight		Maintain a healthy body weight		pp.146–48	
Smoking		Quit smoking		pp.150–51	

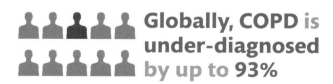

Globally, COPD is under-diagnosed by up to 93%

Taking the test

A clip is placed over your nose. The clinician then asks you to exhale as hard and fast as you can three times into a mouthpiece connected to the spirometer. Repetition is needed to get a reliable reading, because the results are dependent on exactly how you exhale. The test may be done again in 15 minutes after a dose of inhaled medication.

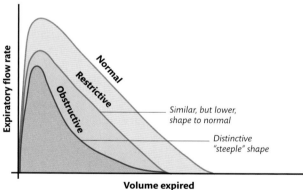

Flow-rate curve
Sometimes the clinician will look at the pattern of flow rate during breathing out. The shapes produced help to distinguish between restrictive and obstructive disorders.

What the results mean

The test measures your breathing rate over the course of one exhalation. Your results are presented as graphs and compared to those predicted for someone of your age, gender, and height. This reveals whether your airways are normal, obstructed, restricted, or a combination. Obstruction could be due to asthma or COPD, which narrow the airways. Inhaled medication often improves the result. Restriction could be due to obesity or kyphoscoliosis – a spine abnormality that prevents the lungs from moving normally.

Lung volume

The most accurate method of measuring lung volume is whole-body plethysmography. Like spirometry (see pp.46–47), it measures the volume of air inhaled and exhaled. However, since the test takes place in a closed box, technicians can determine the volume remaining in the lungs after exhalation, which allows them to calculate total lung capacity (TLC) – the total space inside your lungs that air can occupy.

What the test involves
Whole-body plethysmography takes 3–5 minutes. You sit in a clear booth and a technician supervises you. Pipes are attached to the booth to measure the pressure inside and are connected to a monitor. You are given a mouthpiece and nose clip and are asked to breathe normally, then to pant rapidly while the mouthpiece shutter is closed, and then to breathe as deeply as possible, both in and out. Wear loose, comfortable clothing and avoid smoking for 6 hours beforehand. If you use an inhaler, you may have to stop 6 hours before the test.

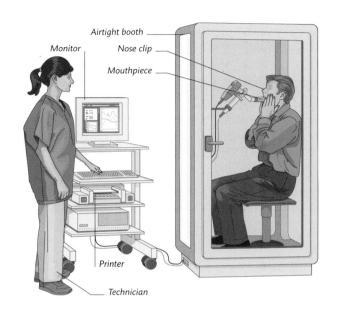

Undergoing the test
You may be asked to hold your cheeks as you breathe to avoid changes in pressure in the mouth due to blowing the cheeks out. You can open the booth from inside if necessary.

Your residual volume is around **1 litre** (2 pints) of "dead air" in your lungs that you cannot exhale

Breathing pattern
This graph shows the pattern of airflow during the test. When you are asked to pant, the mouthpiece shutter is closed. No air flows, but the volume and pressure in your lungs still change. The technicians measure pressure changes in the booth, which allows them to calculate your TLC.

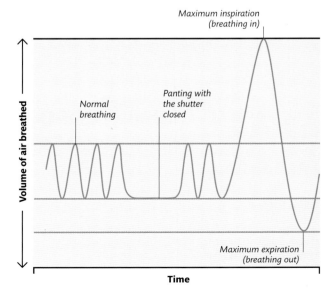

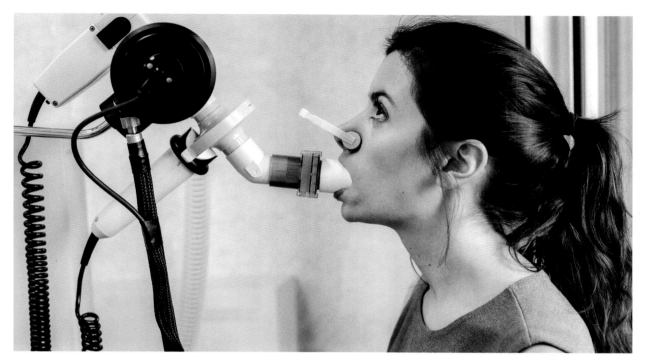

Breathing into a mouthpiece
Whole-body plethysmography uses a mouthpiece similar to spirometry (see pp.46–47). The key difference is that you sit inside an airtight booth, which means that volume changes in your lungs can be measured as changes in air pressure within the booth.

What do the results mean?

The test yields several volume figures in addition to TLC. Tidal volume is the amount of air moved during normal breathing. Inspiratory and expiratory reserve volumes are the additional amounts of air moved during forced breathing. The residual volume is the air remaining in the lungs even after maximum expiration. All these measures can be compared to healthy individuals of the same age, ethnicity, gender, and height. This helps to diagnose obstructive or restrictive lung disease, or both. Causes of restrictive disease include pulmonary fibrosis and obesity. In an obstructive disease, the lungs cannot allow as much air to leave as normal. COPD (chronic obstructive pulmonary disease) and asthma are examples.

Results

Results show four different volume measurements. Each may be of interest, but together they add up to your total lung capacity (TLC).

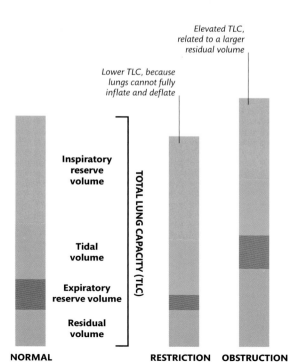

Elevated TLC, related to a larger residual volume

Lower TLC, because lungs cannot fully inflate and deflate

Inspiratory reserve volume

Tidal volume

Expiratory reserve volume

Residual volume

TOTAL LUNG CAPACITY (TLC)

NORMAL　　　　**RESTRICTION**　**OBSTRUCTION**

Exercise capacity

Tests are sometimes needed to measure your heart function, lung function, and blood circulation in response to exercise. They are often used before a major operation, especially to your chest and abdomen, or if you have unexplained breathlessness or chest pain and other tests have been normal.

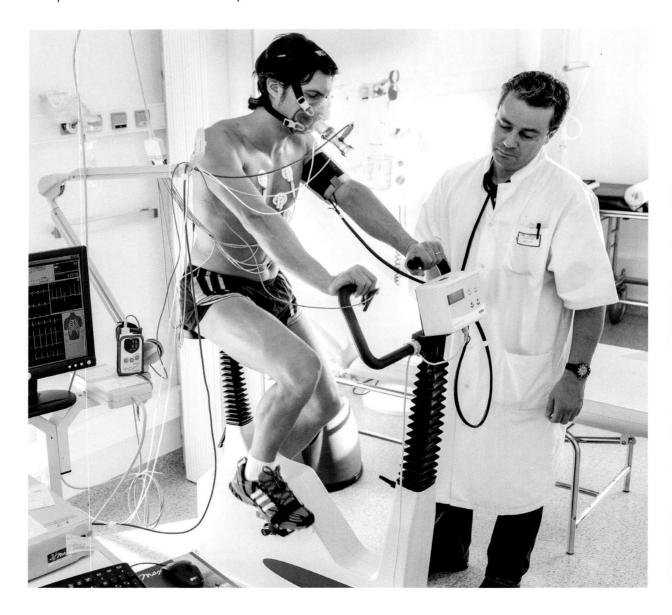

What the test involves

During cardiopulmonary exercise (CPEX) testing, you are instructed to sit on a stationary bicycle. As you pedal, resistance is increased gradually from zero, so that the exercise intensifies. The test can also be done with a treadmill. The results are compared to those expected for someone of your age, sex, and weight. A result lower than expected suggests your fitness is low. This helps your clinician decide whether the proposed surgery is safe. Alternatively, the spirometry, ECG, and oximetry data may identify the cause of your symptoms.

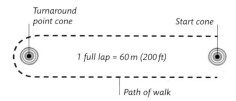

Turnaround point cone

Start cone

1 full lap = 60 m (200 ft)

Path of walk

Walking tests

Other forms of exercise capacity tests include the six-minute walk, in which you walk between two cones and your heart rate and oxygen saturation are monitored. In a variation called the shuttle test, you are asked to walk faster each time until you reach your limit.

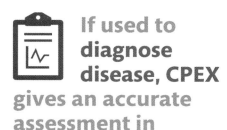

If used to diagnose disease, CPEX gives an accurate assessment in 73–90% of cases

Cardiopulmonary exercise (CPEX) testing

In CPEX testing, you are given a mouthpiece, which measures how much air you breathe (see spirometry, p.47). Chest electrodes record your ECG (see p.37), and an oximeter on your finger (see right) records oxygen saturation.

Blood oxygenation

Pulse oximetry is a painless method of checking how much oxygen is in your blood. The oxygen is attached to the chemical haemoglobin inside red blood cells, which circulate in the bloodstream. The test is performed during a routine examination, or sometimes on arrival at an emergency department.

What the test involves

A plastic device is clipped onto the end of your finger. It shines red and infrared light into your small blood vessels and measures how the light is absorbed, which relates to the oxygen saturation level of the haemoglobin. The result is given as a percentage. The normal range for an adult or child is 95–100 per cent. At 94 per cent or below, you could have an underlying breathing problem such as asthma, or you could simply be very cold and the tracing is not picking up accurately.

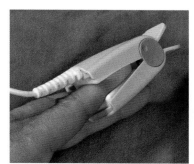

Vital signs
The red light used by oximetry measurement is visible in this portable pulse oximeter, which can be used at your doctor's surgery or in the home. In hospital, pulse oximeters are attached to larger "vital signs" machines that also measure heart rate and blood pressure.

TESTING AT HOME

Most people do not need to monitor their blood oxygenation with a pulse oximeter at home. However, some fitness tracker devices and smart watches shine light through the skin to measure oxygen saturation. Some smartphone apps even use light from your phone's camera flash. However, at present, these are not accurate enough to be trusted as medical devices.

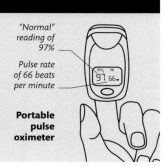

"Normal" reading of 97%

Pulse rate of 66 beats per minute

Portable pulse oximeter

The roles of blood

Blood is the fluid that circulates in the blood vessels to carry oxygen, nutrients, and body chemicals to the cells, and to take waste products away for excretion. The blood is also a vital part of our immune system, which defends the body against disease.

What is in blood?
Blood consists of a liquid called plasma, together with blood cells. Red blood cells carry oxygen from the lungs to body cells. White blood cells fight infection. Platelets are cell fragments that form clots to seal wounds. Plasma carries water, hormones, nutrients, and other chemicals to body tissues and removes waste. It also carries vital proteins, such as immunoglobulins (antibodies) that protect the body from infections.

Red blood cells
Red blood cells contain a red pigment called haemoglobin, which picks up oxygen in the lungs and releases it in the body's cells.

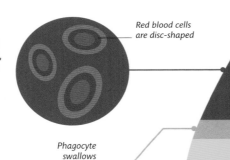

Red blood cells are disc-shaped

45% red blood cells

1% white blood cells and platelets

54% plasma

Phagocyte swallows invaders

White blood cells
The many types of white blood cells, including phagocytes and lymphocytes (B cells and T cells), fight infection and remove harmful substances.

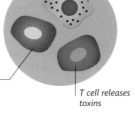

B cell produces antibodies

T cell releases toxins

Antibody

Plasma
Plasma carries antibodies, hormones and other body chemicals, salts and minerals, and water to body tissues. It also removes waste and excess water.

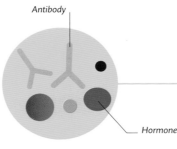

Blood makes up 7–8 per cent of our total body weight

Hormone

The immune system

White blood cells defend the body against pathogens (bacteria, viruses, or other microorganisms), toxins, and cancer cells. There are several types. Phagocytes kill and ingest infectious organisms and dead cells. B cells produce antibodies to stick to targets and mark them for destruction by other white blood cells. T cells destroy infected and cancerous cells. After an infection, some B and T cells "remember" the invading organism in case of another attack.

In some disorders, however, the immune system over-reacts, as in allergies, where it attacks harmless foreign substances, or autoimmune disorders, in which it attacks normal body tissues. Conversely, in immunodeficiency disorders such as AIDS, the system fails to protect the body.

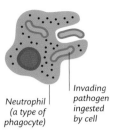

Neutrophil (a type of phagocyte)

Invading pathogen ingested by cell

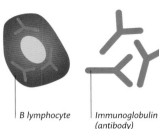

B lymphocyte

Immunoglobulin (antibody)

Destroying pathogens
Neutrophils (above), the most common type of white blood cell, ingest pathogens and damaged tissue.

Producing antibodies
B lymphocytes, or B cells, release antibodies into the plasma. Some B cells recognize pathogens if they re-enter the body.

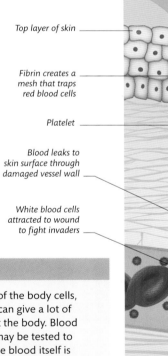

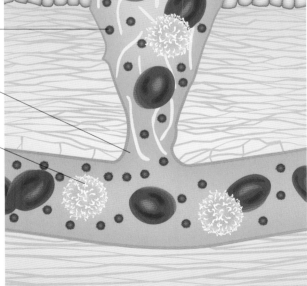

Top layer of skin

Fibrin creates a mesh that traps red blood cells

Platelet

Blood leaks to skin surface through damaged vessel wall

White blood cells attracted to wound to fight invaders

BLOOD TESTS

Blood reaches all of the body cells, so tests on blood can give a lot of information about the body. Blood cells and plasma may be tested to assess how well the blood itself is functioning. Tests on plasma can reveal levels of substances such as glucose and cholesterol, and chemicals produced by the kidneys and the liver. Tests on white blood cells and immunoglobulins can reveal problems with the immune system.

Clotting
When a blood vessel is torn, platelets clump around the injury. The platelets and damaged tissues release chemicals that react with proteins in the plasma called clotting factors, causing a mesh of sticky material (fibrin) to form and trap blood cells, creating a clot. Some blood tests measure platelets and clotting factors to detect whether the blood is clotting properly.

Giving a blood sample

Blood tests are useful for investigating a wide range of conditions and are very commonly performed. For example, you may have a blood test to see if you have a problem such as diabetes, thyroid disease, or an infection; to assess your general health; or to check the health of specific organs, such as the kidneys. Blood tests may also be used to monitor conditions and find out if treatment has been successful.

FINGER-PRICK TESTING

A blood sample can be obtained at home using a finger-pricking technique. The blood can then be sent to a laboratory for testing. If you have diabetes, finger-pricking is a common way of obtaining blood for monitoring your blood glucose levels.

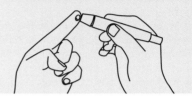

Having a sample taken

Having a blood test is a simple procedure that takes less than five minutes. A tourniquet or tight band is put around your upper arm, which makes the vein swell so that it is easier for the sample to be taken. You may be asked to clench and unclench your fist. A sterile needle, attached to a syringe or a special vacuum container, is inserted into your vein, and a sample of blood is withdrawn. After the sample has been taken, the tourniquet is released and the needle removed. You will be asked to press on the site with a cotton pad, and a small adhesive dressing may be applied. You may get a small bruise but this will fade within a few days. The sample will be sent to the laboratory for analysis. For some blood tests, you may need to fast beforehand. This means you should not eat or drink anything, apart from water, for 8–12 hours before the test. You may also need to stop taking certain medications; if so, your medical professional will let you know.

Obtaining a blood sample

A blood sample is usually taken from a vein in your upper arm. If you tend to feel faint at the sight of blood or needles, you should tell the healthcare professional beforehand so that he or she can try to make you feel more comfortable.

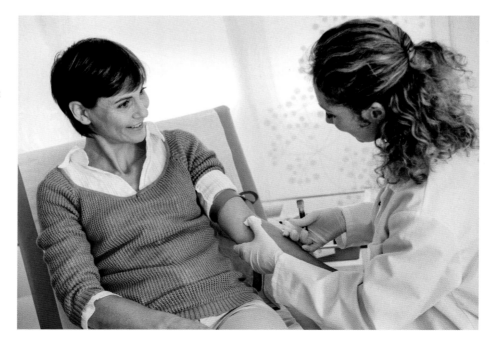

Blood count

A full blood count (FBC) is one of the most common blood tests. Also sometimes known as a complete blood count (CBC), it gives information about red blood cells, white blood cells, and platelets.

What does the test involve?

A blood sample is taken, as described opposite, and the sample is analysed in a laboratory to measure the number of red blood cells, white blood cells, and platelets. Also measured are the size of the red blood cells, the amount of haemoglobin (see pp.52–53) in the red blood cells, and the proportion of blood that comprises red blood cells (known as the haematocrit). If any abnormalities are found, your doctor may recommend further tests to determine the cause or treatment.

WHAT THE RESULTS MIGHT MEAN

Test	Result	Possible cause
Red blood cell levels	Low	Too few red blood cells is most commonly due to iron-deficiency anaemia, which may have various underlying causes, including too little iron in the diet, poor absorption of iron, bleeding, or low levels of folate, vitamin B6, or vitamin B12.
	High	A high level of red blood cells is normal in people who live at high altitude. In other cases, it may be due to smoking, or various disorders, such as the lung disease chronic obstructive pulmonary disease (COPD), kidney disease, or certain blood cancers; it may also be genetic.
Red blood cell size	Abnormally small	The presence of small red blood cells is known as microcytosis. Possible causes include bleeding, iron deficiency, or some genetic disorders, such as the blood disorder thalassaemia.
	Abnormally large	The presence of large red blood cells is termed macrocytosis. Possible causes include thyroid disease, liver disease, or deficiency of vitamin B12.
Haemoglobin level	Low	A low haemoglobin level is a sign of anaemia.
	High	A high haemoglobin level is normal for people who live at high altitude. It may also be due to dehydration, smoking, or an underlying disorder, such as cardiovascular or lung disease.
Haematocrit (proportion of red blood cells in blood)	Low	A low haematocrit reading is a sign of anaemia.
	High	A high haematocrit reading may be the result of dehydration, or it may be due to an underlying disorder, such as lung disease, heart disease, or certain blood disorders.
White blood cell levels	Low	Low white blood cell levels are normal in some people; in others, possible causes include certain infections, such as HIV; blood disorders, such as leukaemia; or certain medications, such as some chemotherapy drugs.
	High	A high white blood cell count is often due to infection. Other possible causes include certain medications, such as corticosteroids; inflammation; severe allergy; stress; and certain blood disorders, such as leukaemia.
Platelet levels	Low	Too few platelets is known as thrombocytopenia. Possible causes include bleeding; certain medications, such as some diuretics; some autoimmune disorders; and bone or blood cancers.
	High	Too many platelets is known as thrombocytosis. Possible causes include acute bleeding; inflammation; infection; removal of the spleen; or disorders such as disease of the bone marrow or certain cancers.

Checking blood glucose

Glucose, a type of sugar, is the primary energy source of all body cells. It is obtained from carbohydrates in the diet and is circulated around the body in the blood. Maintaining the correct blood glucose level is essential for proper functioning of the body. Too high a level indicates diabetes.

Blood glucose control
The level of glucose in the blood is kept within normal limits by various hormones. If the level rises too high – after eating, for example – the pancreas releases insulin to lower the level. If the blood glucose level falls too low, other hormones (such as glucagon from the pancreas) can raise the level by mobilizing carbohydrate stores in the body. If your blood glucose is persistently raised, the cause is either insulin resistance (cells become less responsive to insulin) or decreased production of insulin by the pancreas, indicating diabetes.

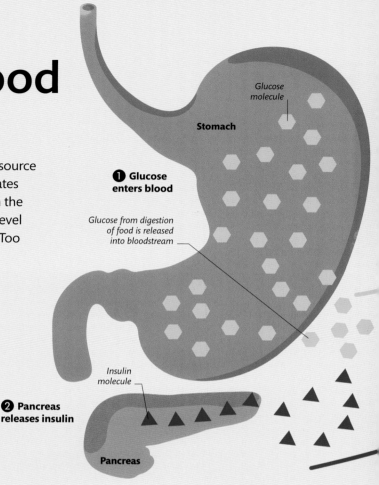

Glucose molecule

Stomach

❶ **Glucose enters blood**

Glucose from digestion of food is released into bloodstream

Insulin molecule

❷ **Pancreas releases insulin**

Pancreas

HbA1c test
Also known as the glycosylated haemoglobin test, the HbA1c test provides a measure of your average blood glucose level over the previous few months. In the blood, glucose joins to haemoglobin (the oxygen-carrying component of blood), forming glycosylated haemoglobin, or HbA1c. The level of HbA1c is not significantly affected by recent food intake, so it provides a good overall picture of your longer-term blood glucose levels. The HbA1C test itself simply involves giving a blood sample (see p.54) for analysis.

HbA1c levels
The blood levels of HbA1c may be given in terms of its concentration (mmol/mol) or what percentage of the blood's haemoglobin is in the form of HbA1c. A level under 42 mmol/mol (5.7 per cent) is considered normal.

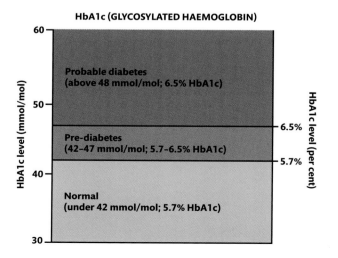

HbA1c (GLYCOSYLATED HAEMOGLOBIN)

HbA1c level (mmol/mol)

HbA1c level (per cent)

60 —

**Probable diabetes
(above 48 mmol/mol; 6.5% HbA1c)**

50 —

— 6.5%

**Pre-diabetes
(42–47 mmol/mol; 5.7–6.5% HbA1c)**

— 5.7%

40 —

**Normal
(under 42 mmol/mol; 5.7% HbA1c)**

30 —

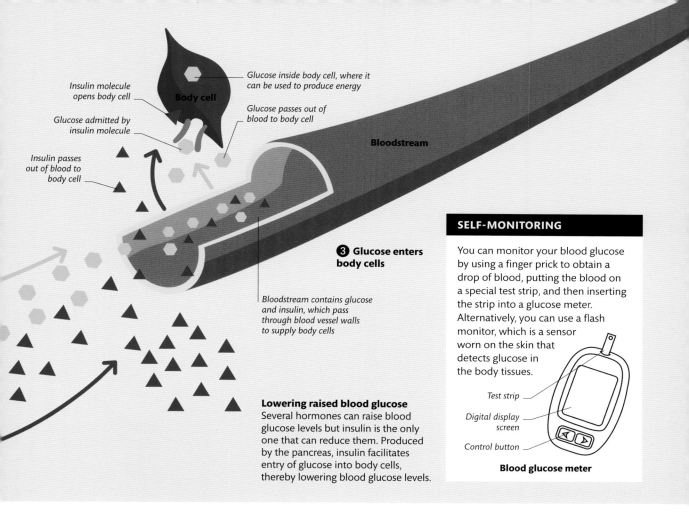

Insulin molecule opens body cell

Glucose admitted by insulin molecule

Insulin passes out of blood to body cell

Body cell

Glucose inside body cell, where it can be used to produce energy

Glucose passes out of blood to body cell

Bloodstream

③ Glucose enters body cells

Bloodstream contains glucose and insulin, which pass through blood vessel walls to supply body cells

Lowering raised blood glucose
Several hormones can raise blood glucose levels but insulin is the only one that can reduce them. Produced by the pancreas, insulin facilitates entry of glucose into body cells, thereby lowering blood glucose levels.

SELF-MONITORING

You can monitor your blood glucose by using a finger prick to obtain a drop of blood, putting the blood on a special test strip, and then inserting the strip into a glucose meter. Alternatively, you can use a flash monitor, which is a sensor worn on the skin that detects glucose in the body tissues.

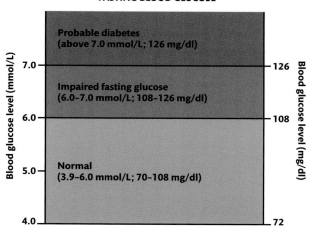

Test strip

Digital display screen

Control button

Blood glucose meter

Fasting blood glucose

This test involves checking your blood glucose level after you have not eaten for several hours. It provides an accurate measure of your general blood glucose level because the result is not influenced by anything you may have eaten. You will be instructed not to eat for 8–10 hours before the test and also to avoid drinking anything apart from normal or small amounts of plain water. You can usually continue to take most medications but you should ask your health professional if you are not sure. After the fasting period, a blood sample is taken in the usual way (see p.54) and the amount of glucose in the sample is measured.

Fasting blood glucose levels
The blood glucose level after fasting can indicate whether you have diabetes or impaired fasting glucose (a type of pre-diabetes).

FASTING BLOOD GLUCOSE

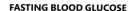

Blood glucose level (mmol/L)

Blood glucose level (mg/dl)

**Probable diabetes
(above 7.0 mmol/L; 126 mg/dl)**

7.0 — 126

**Impaired fasting glucose
(6.0–7.0 mmol/L; 108–126 mg/dl)**

6.0 — 108

**Normal
(3.9–6.0 mmol/L; 70–108 mg/dl)**

5.0

4.0 — 72

Checking blood cholesterol

Cholesterol is a fat-like substance carried in the blood. Some cholesterol is vital for normal functioning of the body but too much of a certain type may increase your risk of developing health problems such heart disease and stroke.

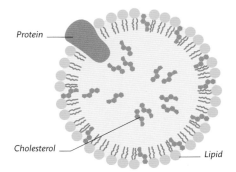

"BAD" CHOLESTEROL

Protein

Cholesterol

Lipid

What does cholesterol do?

Cholesterol plays a vital role in many body functions, such as making hormones, producing bile to help digestion, and keeping cell membranes flexible but firm. About 90 per cent of cholesterol in the body is made in the liver; only a small proportion comes from the diet. Cholesterol is carried in your blood attached to proteins, in particles called lipoproteins. There are two main types of these: low-density lipoproteins (LDLs) and high-density lipoproteins (HDLs). Triglycerides are another type of fat in the bloodstream. When you eat more calories (energy) than you need, the excess energy is converted into triglycerides by the liver then stored in body cells. High blood levels of triglycerides are associated with an increased risk of cardiovascular disease, which is why it is important to measure blood levels of triglycerides as well as cholesterol.

Low-density lipoprotein (LDL)

Containing a relatively small amount of protein and large amount of cholesterol, LDL particles carry cholesterol from the liver to the body cells. LDL can deposit cholesterol on artery walls, forming fatty plaques that reduce blood flow, which is why LDL is called "bad" cholesterol.

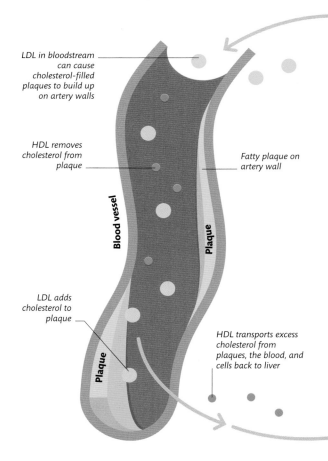

LDL in bloodstream can cause cholesterol-filled plaques to build up on artery walls

HDL removes cholesterol from plaque

Fatty plaque on artery wall

Blood vessel

Plaque

LDL adds cholesterol to plaque

Plaque

HDL transports excess cholesterol from plaques, the blood, and cells back to liver

---

HOME CHOLESTEROL TESTS

You can check your cholesterol yourself with a home testing kit. This uses a special reactive strip on which you place a drop of blood from a finger prick. The strip is then inserted into an analyser, which gives the results within a few minutes. As well as the total cholesterol level, some devices also measure HDL, LDL, and triglyceride levels and calculate the HDL to LDL ratio. Alternatively, there are home tests in which you send off the strip or a blood sample to a laboratory for analysis. Some pharmacies also offer blood cholesterol tests. The results should be considered in combination with other risk factors for cardiovascular disease, and appropriate medical advice should be sought.

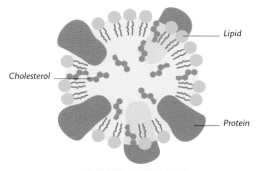

"GOOD" CHOLESTEROL

Lipid

Cholesterol

Protein

High-density lipoprotein (HDL)
HDL particles contain relatively more protein and less cholesterol than LDLs. HDL helps to remove cholesterol from fatty plaques on the artery walls and carries the cholesterol to the liver for removal from the body, which is why HDL is known as "good" cholesterol.

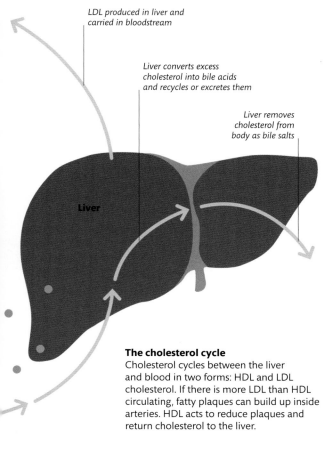

LDL produced in liver and carried in bloodstream

Liver converts excess cholesterol into bile acids and recycles or excretes them

Liver removes cholesterol from body as bile salts

Liver

The cholesterol cycle
Cholesterol cycles between the liver and blood in two forms: HDL and LDL cholesterol. If there is more LDL than HDL circulating, fatty plaques can build up inside arteries. HDL acts to reduce plaques and return cholesterol to the liver.

Measuring cholesterol levels
Cholesterol levels are measured by analysing blood obtained from a finger prick or by taking a small sample from a vein in the arm (see p.54). You may sometimes, but not always, be asked to fast for 8–12 hours before the blood sample is taken. If you are asked to fast, you should not eat or drink anything, apart from plain water. You may also be asked to stop taking certain medications; if in doubt, consult your health professional. The blood sample is analysed for HDL and LDL cholesterol levels, and often also for triglycerides. The HDL and LDL levels enable the total cholesterol and the total to HDL ratio to be calculated. Together, the results give an indication of your cardiovascular health in relation to your blood lipid level.

BLOOD LIPID LEVELS		
Total cholesterol (mmol/L; mg/dl)	*Total cholesterol: HDL ratio*	*Triglyceride (mmol/L; mg/dl)*
Unhealthy Above 5 mmol/L (195 mg/dl)	**Unhealthy** Above 4	**Unhealthy** Above 2.3 mmol/L (205 mg/dl) (non-fasting blood test) Above 1.7 mmol/L (150 mg/dl) (fasting blood test)
Healthy Below 5 mmol/L (195 mg/dl)	**Healthy** Below 4, ideally as low as possible	**Healthy** Below 2.3 mmol/L (205 mg/dl) (non-fasting blood test) Below 1.7 mmol/L (150 mg/dl) (fasting blood test)

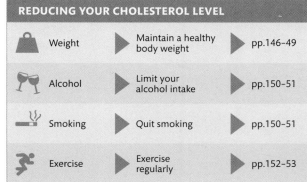

REDUCING YOUR CHOLESTEROL LEVEL				
	Weight	Maintain a healthy body weight		pp.146–49
	Alcohol	Limit your alcohol intake		pp.150–51
	Smoking	Quit smoking		pp.150–51
	Exercise	Exercise regularly		pp.152–53

Other blood tests

Blood may be tested for more than 100 different substances. Some tests are carried out only to diagnose specific health problems, while others, such as liver function tests, are widely used for both diagnosis and health checking.

Automated blood testing
Most blood samples are analysed automatically by machine, which produces quick, accurate results. The results are then evaluated by a medical professional.

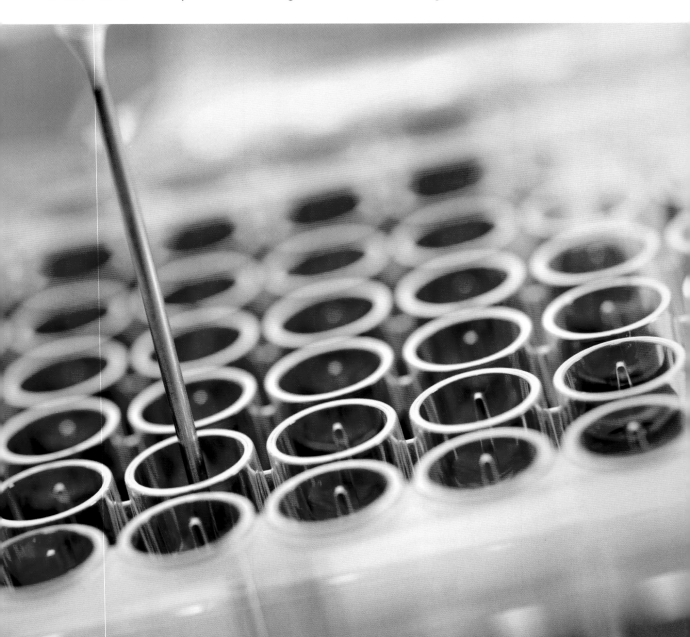

Types of blood tests

As well as checking the levels of blood cells (see p.55) and substances such as glucose (see pp.56–57) and cholesterol (see pp.58–59), blood can be tested for numerous other substances, including vitamins, minerals, proteins, hormones, enzymes, antibodies, and even certain genes. The table below lists some of the more common tests and what the results may indicate.

Test	What is measured/detected	What the results might mean
Vitamins and minerals	Calcium (an essential mineral)	Abnormal levels of calcium may indicate a health problem, such as parathyroid disease, kidney disease, a bone disorder, or certain cancers.
	Phosphate (an essential mineral)	Abnormal phosphate levels may be due to various health problems, including kidney problems, parathyroid gland problems, excessive vitamin D, or cancer.
	Vitamin B12 and folate	Low levels of these substances may indicate anaemia, too little dietary intake of the substances, or autoimmune disease; certain medications may also cause low levels.
	Vitamin D	Low levels of this vitamin may be due to various causes, including dietary deficiency, too little exposure to sunlight, impaired kidney function, or certain disorders that impair absorption in the intestine, such as coeliac disease.
	Ferritin (a form of iron stored in the body)	Low levels of ferritin usually indicate anaemia. High ferritin levels may indicate any of various underlying disorders, such as liver disease, diabetes, or some types of cancer; obesity may also cause high ferritin levels.
Blood clotting	Clotting factors (proteins essential for normal clotting)	Abnormal levels of clotting factors may indicate a disorder, such as liver disease or a bleeding disorder. Clotting factor levels are also used to monitor treatment with some anticoagulant drugs.
Infection and inflammation	The presence of specific antibodies	The presence of an antibody against a specific infection indicates that you have or have had that infection.
	CRP (C-reactive protein, a substance produced in the liver in response to inflammation)	High levels of CRP indicate the presence of inflammation somewhere in the body; however, this does not indicate what part of the body is inflamed.
Thyroid function tests	Levels of thyroid hormones (thyroid-stimulating hormone, thyroxine, triiodothyronine)	Abnormal thyroid hormone levels may indicate that your thyroid gland is overactive (hyperthyroidism) or underactive (hypothyroidism).
Liver function tests	Levels of certain proteins and liver enzymes	Abnormal levels of liver proteins or enzymes may indicate liver injury. See also p.71.
Kidney function tests	Levels of urea (a waste product of protein metabolism), creatinine (a waste product formed in muscles), and electrolytes	Levels of these substances indicate how well your kidneys are working. High levels of any of these substances may indicate kidney injury. See also p.77.
Cancer tests	Prostate-specific antigen (PSA) – a protein associated with prostate problems	High levels of PSA may indicate a prostate problem, such as an enlarged or inflamed prostate or prostate cancer. However, PSA levels may be abnormal without there being an underlying problem.
	CA-125 protein	High CA-125 levels may indicate various reproductive system problems in women, including ovarian cancer and ovarian cysts. However, high levels may also occur normally, during menstruation, for example.
	BRCA1 and BRCA2 genes	The presence of certain versions of these genes is associated with an increased risk of breast and ovarian cancer.

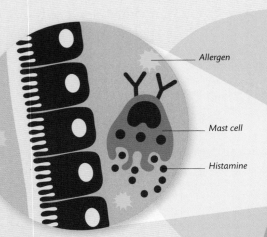

Allergen

Mast cell

Histamine

COMMON ALLERGIES

Hayfever (also called allergic rhinitis), eczema, and asthma are among the most common allergies. As with other allergies, they are due to an overreaction of the body's immune system, which produces excessive amounts of substances such as histamine and cytokines. It is these substances that cause the symptoms of allergy.

Sinus

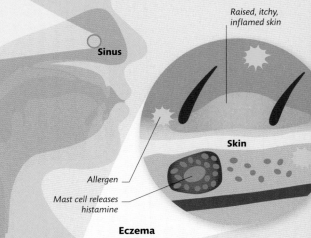

Raised, itchy, inflamed skin

Skin

Allergen

Mast cell releases histamine

Hayfever
Many people suffer from hayfever, or allergic rhinitis, an allergy to pollen or dust. When allergens bind to mast cells (a type of immune cell) just below the lining of the nose, sinuses, and eyes, these cells release histamine. The histamine triggers an inflammatory response, including sneezing, a runny nose, and itchy, watery eyes.

Eczema
Eczema is probably triggered by an irritant (allergen) on the skin that stimulates mast cells in the deeper layers of the skin to release histamine, which causes inflammation and irritation.

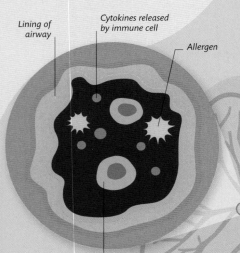

Lining of airway

Cytokines released by immune cell

Allergen

Immune cell

Constricted airway

Cytokine

Lung

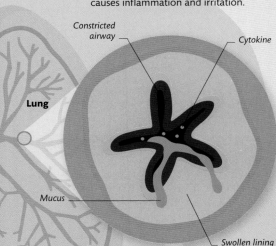

Mucus

Swollen lining of airway

Normal immune response in lungs
When an allergen is inhaled, immune cells in the airways of the lungs produce chemicals called cytokines. Normally, these substances cause only minor swelling of the airways.

Asthma attack
In an asthma attack, there is an exaggerated response to an inhaled allergen. The cytokines cause the airways to swell and produce large amounts of mucus, leading to symptoms including wheezing, coughing, and breathlessness.

Checking for allergies

An allergy is an exaggerated response by the immune system to a substance that is normally harmless, such as a pollen or a specific food. Allergies are not usually serious, although rarely they can be life-threatening. Tests for allergies include skin prick testing and patch testing.

The body's allergic response

The body continually encounters foreign substances that stimulate the immune system. Normally, this does not cause any problems, but in susceptible people the immune system overreacts to a particular substance (the allergen), causing an allergic reaction. Most allergic responses occur shortly after exposure to the allergen, but sometimes a reaction may not occur for up to about three days after exposure. Most people with an allergy have only relatively mild symptoms, such as a runny nose, rash, watering eyes, sneezing, and wheezing. Rarely, a severe allergic response may occur, causing symptoms of anaphylactic shock: swelling of the face, mouth, throat, and tongue, difficulty breathing, and possibly loss of consciousness. Anaphylactic shock is a medical emergency that needs immediate treatment with an injection of adrenaline (epinephrine).

Skin prick testing

Skin prick testing is one of the most common allergy tests and is carried out to identify possible allergens immediately. Dilute solutions are produced from extracts of allergens that commonly cause allergic reactions, such as pollen, foods, and dander (flakes of skin shed from animals). A drop of each solution is placed on your skin, which is then pricked with a needle. The doctor examines the skin for a reaction, which typically occurs within about 10–15 minutes. If you are allergic to one of the test substances, an inflamed, red, itchy lump appears. The size of the lump is not an indication of how severe your allergy is. If you usually take antihistamines or other anti-allergy medications, you may need to stop taking them for a few days before testing, depending on the specific medication.

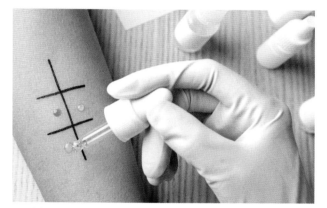

Applying drops of possible allergens

Patch testing

Patch testing is used to investigate contact dermatitis, a type of allergic eczema. It is carried out to determine which substances provoke your eczema. Tiny amounts of possible allergens are placed on small patches or metal discs, which are then taped to your skin. They are commonly taped to your back, but sometimes your arms or legs may be used instead. After about two days, the patches or discs are removed and the skin underneath is examined by a dermatologist. A red, itchy, inflamed area indicates a positive reaction to the particular allergen on the patch or disc. The dermatologist will re-examine the test area about two days later to check for any delayed reactions. If you usually take anti-allergy medication, you will be asked to stop taking it before the test.

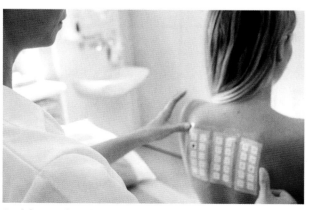

Applying patches of possible allergens

Your digestive system

The digestive system breaks down food and drink to release nutrients and energy for body cells. It is centred on a long tube called the alimentary canal. It also includes the liver, gallbladder, and pancreas, which supply digestive chemicals.

The alimentary canal
The distinct parts of the alimentary canal carry out the digestion and absorption of food and drink in several stages. The material remaining at the end of these processes is expelled as faeces.

Mouth and oesophagus
Food is broken down physically by the teeth and chemically by an enzyme called amylase in the saliva. The tongue mixes the food and saliva to form a ball (bolus) for swallowing. This passes down the gullet (oesophagus) to the stomach.

Stomach
Food is mixed with strong stomach acids and enzymes and churned by the muscular stomach walls, so that it breaks down into a semi-liquid substance called chyme. Food may stay in the stomach for hours before entering the intestine.

Small intestine
This long, muscular tube has three sections. In the first and second sections (duodenum and jejunum), food is mixed with further digestive juices to release nutrients. In the third (ileum), the nutrients are absorbed into the blood and lymph.

Large intestine (colon)
This tube contains bacteria that act on the remains of the food to release further nutrients. The large intestine also absorbs water into the body. The remaining waste is concentrated to form faeces, which pass out via the rectum and anus.

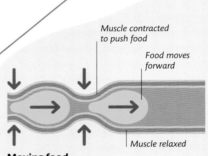

Muscle contracted to push food

Food moves forward

Muscle relaxed

Moving food
Boluses of food are pushed along the digestive tract by wave-like contractions of the muscle walls in the oesophagus and intestines. This action is called peristalsis.

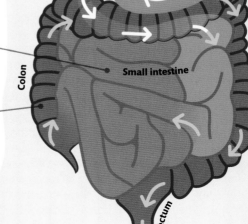

Nasal cavity

Mouth

Oesophagus

Stomach

Colon

Small intestine

Rectum

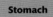

The **intestinal lining** is about **32 sq m** (345 sq ft) in area – or around **eight kingsize beds**

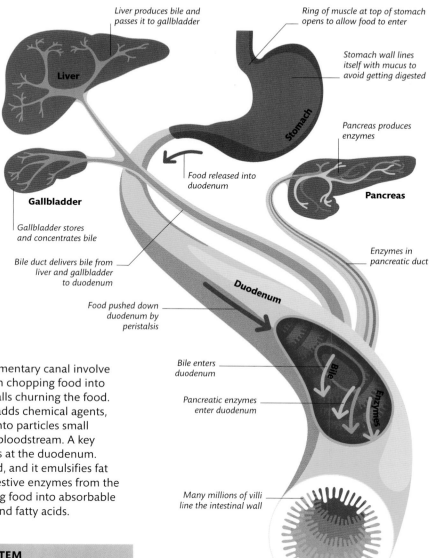

Liver produces bile and passes it to gallbladder

Liver

Ring of muscle at top of stomach opens to allow food to enter

Stomach wall lines itself with mucus to avoid getting digested

Stomach

Pancreas produces enzymes

Food released into duodenum

Gallbladder

Pancreas

Gallbladder stores and concentrates bile

Bile duct delivers bile from liver and gallbladder to duodenum

Enzymes in pancreatic duct

Duodenum

Food pushed down duodenum by peristalsis

Bile enters duodenum

Bile

Pancreatic enzymes enter duodenum

Enzymes

Many millions of villi line the intestinal wall

Digesting food

The digestive processes in the alimentary canal involve physical actions, such as the teeth chopping food into small pieces, and the stomach walls churning the food. However, throughout, the body adds chemical agents, mainly enzymes, to digest food into particles small enough to be absorbed into the bloodstream. A key cocktail of these chemicals enters at the duodenum. Bile from the gallbladder is added, and it emulsifies fat into tiny droplets. A range of digestive enzymes from the pancreas also enter here, breaking food into absorbable nutrients – sugars, amino acids, and fatty acids.

TESTS ON THE DIGESTIVE SYSTEM

Tests may be carried out to assess the digestive system structures, or the levels of digestive enzymes and other chemicals. Imaging such as X-rays, or viewing with endoscopy, can reveal blocked or narrowed areas, tumours, or bleeding in the digestive tract. Certain tests are done to detect ulcers (sore areas in the stomach or duodenum lining). Blood tests may be carried out to assess the levels of chemicals produced by the liver, or of insulin or digestive enzymes from the pancreas.

Intestinal lining

The lining of the small intestine is covered with millions of tiny, finger-like structures called villi. These, in turn, are covered with smaller microvilli. The villi provide a huge surface area to enable nutrients to be absorbed into the blood.

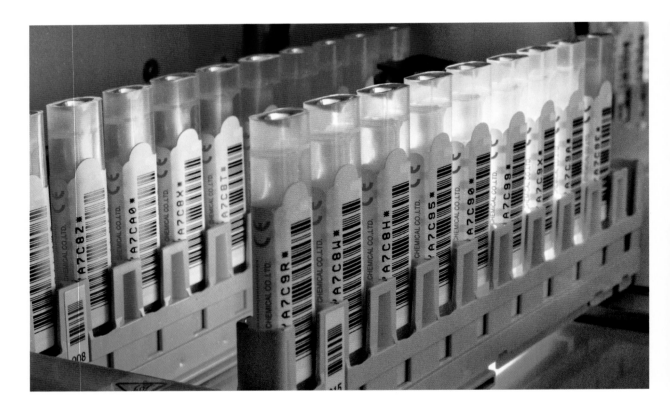

Automated test
Specimen tubes sit in a machine that automatically carries out faecal immunochemical tests (FIT) to look for the presence of blood in the samples.

Screening for bowel cancer

Bowel or colorectal cancer is common worldwide, mostly affecting those over the age of 50. Screening tests are designed to identify early-stage cancers, which have a better chance of being effectively treated.

FAECAL BLOOD TESTS
There are two tests that look for non-visible blood in stool, which could be a sign of bowel cancer.

How the tests are done
The faecal occult blood test (FOB) and the faecal immunochemical test (FIT) both require a faecal sample. The FOB test requires the user to collect a stool on three separate occasions and wipe a small amount onto the enclosed card. The FIT only requires one sample, which is collected on a stick and put into a plastic tube. Follow the instruction carefully to ensure accuracy.

What the results mean
The results may be: normal (no blood noted in the stool), which will require no immediate action; unclear, which would require a repeat test; or abnormal (blood found in sample). An abnormal result may or may not be caused by bowel cancer; in this case you would be invited to have a colonoscopy (so that the lining of the colon can be viewed).

BOWEL SCOPE SCREENING

Bowel scope screening uses a technique called flexible sigmoidoscopy. A thin flexible tube with a camera is inserted into the bowel to identify and remove polyps that could turn into cancer over time.

What the test involves

The test takes place in a hospital or clinic. Information about the test and an enema or strong laxative to clear the bowels are sent to your home address beforehand. You may be advised on dietary changes to make prior to the test and you will need to use the laxative on the day of the test to enable the bowel to be clear as possible. During the test the camera is inserted into the rectum and moved into the sigmoid colon, after which some air is used to inflate the bowel. If any polyps are found, a sample would usually be removed during the same procedure. The bowel scope screening is done with the patient awake and it is not usually painful.

What the results may mean

This particular test cannot reach the whole of the bowel, so if some polyps are found, a colonoscopy would usually be offered. Any polyps removed are sent to a laboratory for testing. You will be told that polyps have been sent for analysis on the day of the procedure. If a polyp is found to contain cancerous cells, you would be sent to a cancer specialist for treatment.

The sigmoid or pelvic colon is the S-shaped, last section of the large intestine

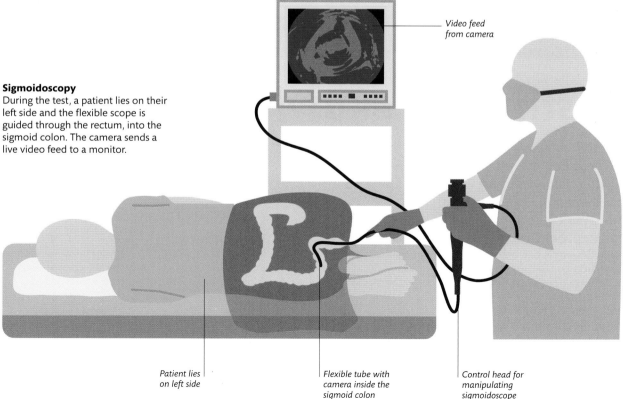

Sigmoidoscopy
During the test, a patient lies on their left side and the flexible scope is guided through the rectum, into the sigmoid colon. The camera sends a live video feed to a monitor.

Video feed from camera

Patient lies on left side

Flexible tube with camera inside the sigmoid colon

Control head for manipulating sigmoidoscope

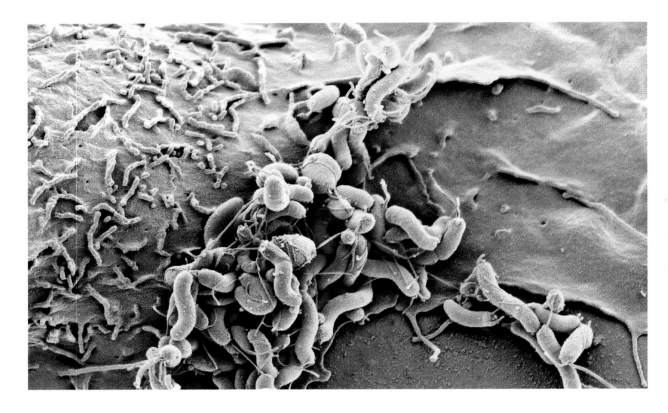

Testing for *H. pylori*

Helicobacter pylori is a type of bacteria that thrives in the stomach lining, where it can cause recurrent indigestion and stomach (gastric) ulcers to develop. It may also be present but cause no symptoms, which is why many people who have the infection are not aware of it.

Bacterial infection
A magnified view shows a number of *H. pylori* bacteria (coloured yellow) on cells from a person's stomach.

FAECAL ANTIGEN TEST
A stool sample can be used to identify an active *H. pylori* infection by checking for antigens (substances that cause an immune response) associated with the bacteria.

What the test involves
A stool sample is sent to the lab for analysis. You do not need to fast before the stool sample is given, but you will need to avoid taking any antibiotics for a month beforehand as they may affect *H. pylori* bacteria. Acid-suppressing medication can't be taken for the two weeks before the sample is given.

What the result means
If an active infection is detected, your doctor will prescribe antibiotics. You will also need to be tested again after the treatment to ensure that the infection has been cured.

H. pylori is **found in up to 50 per cent of the population**

BREATH TEST
The presence of *H. pylori* in the stomach can be detected by analysing a breath sample taken after drinking a special liquid.

What the test involves
You will be given a drink that contains urea (which is tasteless), and after waiting 15–30 minutes, a breath sample will be taken. You will need to stop taking antibiotics for four weeks or acid-reducing medication for two weeks leading up to the test, as these could affect the validity of the test result; your doctor or the test centre should give you details. You will also need to fast for six hours before the test.

PREVENTING *H. PYLORI* INFECTIONS

Helicobacter pylori infection is thought to be widespread, though most affected people do not experience any symptoms. It is not completely clear how a person becomes infected with the bacterium. It could be through coming into contact with stools from an infected person, or via food or drink that they have prepared. Good hygiene practices, such as hand washing and eating properly cooked food can help to prevent infection. Recurrence in a partially treated person can also occur, for example if the treatment is not taken properly.

How the test works
Before you swallow the liquid containing the urea you will be asked give a breath sample for a baseline to compare against. If *H. pylori* is present, it will break down the urea solution and this can be detected on your breath.

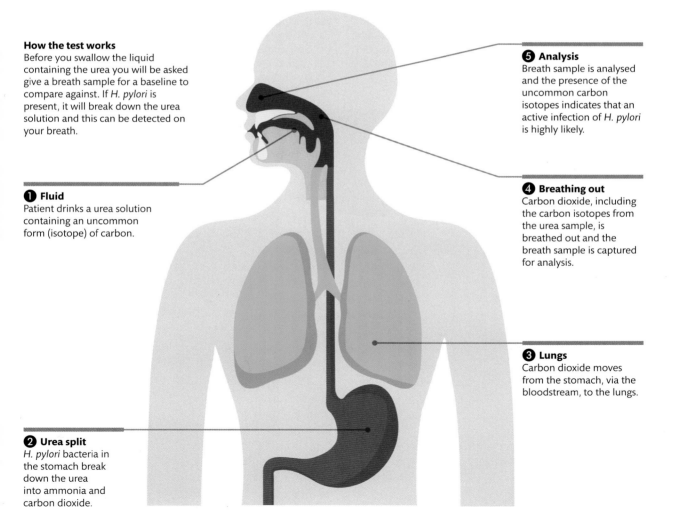

5 Analysis
Breath sample is analysed and the presence of the uncommon carbon isotopes indicates that an active infection of *H. pylori* is highly likely.

1 Fluid
Patient drinks a urea solution containing an uncommon form (isotope) of carbon.

4 Breathing out
Carbon dioxide, including the carbon isotopes from the urea sample, is breathed out and the breath sample is captured for analysis.

3 Lungs
Carbon dioxide moves from the stomach, via the bloodstream, to the lungs.

2 Urea split
H. pylori bacteria in the stomach break down the urea into ammonia and carbon dioxide.

Abdominal ultrasound

An ultrasound of the abdomen is an outpatient test performed at many clinics or hospitals. It is quick, non-invasive, and painless. This scan is performed to enable doctors to view the organs in the abdomen and identify possible causes of abdominal complaints such as pain, bloating, nausea, or vomiting.

What the test involves

The test is performed by a technician who will press a probe, which emits sound waves, onto your abdomen. The echoes of the sound waves allow images to be created of your vital organs, such as the liver, gallbladder, spleen, and kidneys. If you are a man, you may be asked to wear a gown or remove your top clothing. If you are a woman, you will need to wear a front-opening gown. You should not eat or drink anything for a few hours beforehand. The scan usually lasts 10 to 15 minutes.

What the results mean

The images created by the scan may take a few minutes to be interpreted, but if the test is not urgent, you may only get the results a few days later, or at your next doctor's appointment. The scan can detect many health problems, such as gallstones, kidney stones, an enlarged spleen, or a hernia of the abdominal wall.

Sometimes it is not possible to get a clear view of all your abdominal organs. If this happens, your clinician may refer you for another type of scan.

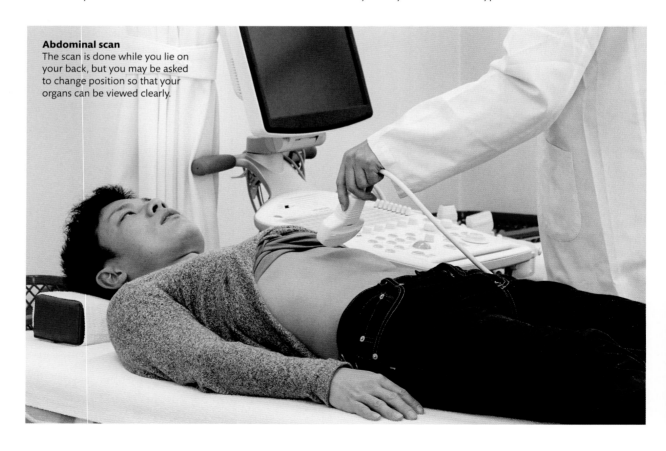

Abdominal scan
The scan is done while you lie on your back, but you may be asked to change position so that your organs can be viewed clearly.

Liver blood tests

Liver blood tests, also sometimes called liver function tests, are done to find out how well your liver is working. They involve measuring the levels of various substances, such as proteins and enzymes, in the blood.

What the test involves
For the tests, you will need to have blood taken (see p.54). Some food and medication may influence the results and you will need to check with your doctor beforehand to see what needs to be avoided prior to the test. The test looks at a number of indicators to diagnose liver issues such as infection, inflammation, or a blockage in the bile ducts. It also measures the liver's ability to produce a protein called albumin and blood-clotting factors. The tests are also done to detect signs of liver disease. Other blood tests that seem unrelated to your liver may be requested at the same time; for example, a full blood count (see p.55).

What the results mean
The blood samples are sent to the lab for analysis and it can take a few hours for the results to be processed. An abnormal result does not necessarily indicate liver disease, and sometimes additional tests will be required. The tests may also be used to monitor the progression of a disease or to monitor the possible side-effects of medication.

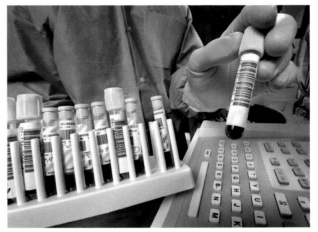

Blood test
The blood sample is analysed to look for any abnormal levels in the enzymes, proteins, and other substances produced by the liver.

What is tested	What this means
Alanine transaminase (ALT)	This is raised when the liver cells are damaged or inflamed.
Aspartate transaminase (AST)	This is raised when cells are damaged or inflamed, but AST is not specific to cells in the liver.
Alkaline phosphatase (ALP)	This is raised when there is a blockage, such as gallstones, within the bile ducts.
Albumin and total protein	Low levels of albumin or total protein mean that your liver is not working properly, and could indicate liver failure. Malnutrition can also cause a lower level of albumin.
Bilirubin	High levels of bilirubin can indicate that there is an obstruction of the bile ducts in your liver or in your gallbladder. It may also indicate liver damage due to inflammation.
γ-Glutamyltransferase (GGT)	Raised when there is damage to your liver. It can also be raised by chronic excess alcohol consumption.
L-lactate dehydrogenase (LD)	This enzyme is released when cells anywhere in the body are damaged or break down. It can be raised in many conditions, such as liver disease, as well limb injury, or haemolytic anaemia.
Prothrombin time (PT)	This measures of how quickly your blood clots. A high prothrombin time means that your liver is adequately producing clotting chemicals and is a sign of liver disease. Medications such as warfarin can also affect this.

Urinary system

The urinary system consists of the kidneys and bladder, plus the urinary vessels – the ureters and urethra – that connect them to the outside world. Blood enters the kidney via the renal artery. It passes through smaller vessels to the nephrons (see below, left) for filtering. Cleaned, filtered blood leaves the kidney via the renal vein. Urine is collected in the renal pelvis and passes into the ureters, where it flows to the bladder for storage prior to urination through the urethra.

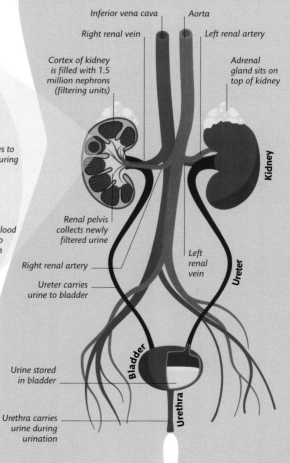

Inferior vena cava
Aorta
Right renal vein
Left renal artery
Cortex of kidney is filled with 1.5 million nephrons (filtering units)
Adrenal gland sits on top of kidney
Renal pelvis collects newly filtered urine
Left renal vein
Right renal artery
Ureter carries urine to bladder
Kidney
Ureter
Urine stored in bladder
Bladder
Urethra carries urine during urination
Urethra

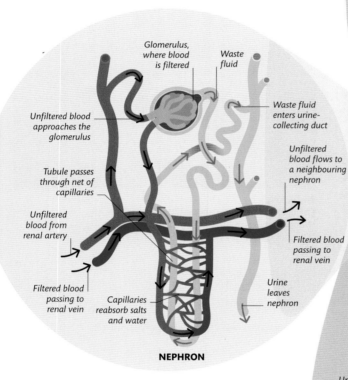

Glomerulus, where blood is filtered
Waste fluid
Unfiltered blood approaches the glomerulus
Waste fluid enters urine-collecting duct
Tubule passes through net of capillaries
Unfiltered blood flows to a neighbouring nephron
Unfiltered blood from renal artery
Filtered blood passing to renal vein
Filtered blood passing to renal vein
Capillaries reabsorb salts and water
Urine leaves nephron

NEPHRON

Filtering the blood

Blood entering the kidney passes through microscopically small filtering units called nephrons. The blood first enters a knot of capillaries (tiny blood vessels) called a glomerulus. Here, waste materials and excess fluid are filtered out of the blood. The filtered fluid passes through looped tubules where essential fluids and substances are reabsorbed into the blood, while the waste leaves the kidneys as urine.

How your kidneys work

The kidneys are a pair of bean-shaped organs midway down your back. As the key components of the urinary system, they have two main jobs: filtering waste products out of the blood and regulating the body's fluid balance.

The kidneys' nephrons and tubules, laid end to end, would stretch 80 km (50 miles)

Fluid balance
The kidneys constantly exchange signals with the endocrine (hormonal) system and the circulatory system (see p.27) to balance the amounts of water, salts, minerals, and waste that are expelled in urine or retained in the bloodstream and body tissues. This is essential as dehydration (having too little fluid in your tissues) can upset vital functions such as regulating blood pressure and body temperature. Having too much fluid is rare but can also pose risks to health.

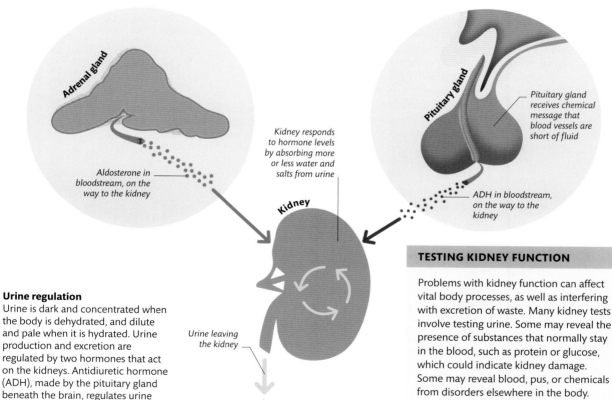

Adrenal gland

Aldosterone in bloodstream, on the way to the kidney

Kidney responds to hormone levels by absorbing more or less water and salts from urine

Kidney

Pituitary gland

Pituitary gland receives chemical message that blood vessels are short of fluid

ADH in bloodstream, on the way to the kidney

Urine leaving the kidney

Urine

Urine concentration controlled by the kidneys

Urine regulation
Urine is dark and concentrated when the body is dehydrated, and dilute and pale when it is hydrated. Urine production and excretion are regulated by two hormones that act on the kidneys. Antidiuretic hormone (ADH), made by the pituitary gland beneath the brain, regulates urine volume. Aldosterone, secreted by the adrenal glands (just above the kidneys), regulates levels of water, sodium, and potassium in the urine.

TESTING KIDNEY FUNCTION
Problems with kidney function can affect vital body processes, as well as interfering with excretion of waste. Many kidney tests involve testing urine. Some may reveal the presence of substances that normally stay in the blood, such as protein or glucose, which could indicate kidney damage. Some may reveal blood, pus, or chemicals from disorders elsewhere in the body. Blood may also be tested, to assess how well your glomeruli are functioning to filter the blood.

Urine analysis

Urine analysis, or urinalysis, encompasses a range of tests performed on a sample of urine. These can be done either during your appointment with a healthcare professional (urine dipstick test) or in the laboratory (urine microscopy and culture) in order to diagnose and monitor a variety of conditions including diabetes, infection, and chronic kidney disease.

Giving a sample
You may be asked to provide a mid-stream, clean catch sample of urine. This means that the first and last parts of your urine stream, which are more likely to be contaminated with bacteria from the skin, are not included in the sample. If you are female, it is best to wash your labia first, and hold the labia open as you collect the sample.

Your doctor or nurse will provide you with a sterile container and this should have your details and the date written clearly on it. A sample can be kept in a fridge for up to 24 hours if you are unable to give it to your doctor within the hour. Urine samples provided first thing in the morning will be more concentrated and therefore more likely to pick up an abnormal result. Urine samples can also be affected by your diet, physical activity, and dehydration, so it is important to mention this to your doctor if you think it may be relevant.

Home testing kits are available, but it is advisable to see your GP or practice nurse to get your urine tested. They will be able to provide the right equipment and have the expertise to interpret the results correctly, and send the sample off for further tests, if needed. You should get your urine tested if you notice blood in the urine, if you are passing urine more often than usual and/or with any pain, burning, or stinging, or if the urine is cloudy, smelly, or a different colour from usual.

Bacteria test
Urine may be sent to a laboratory for analysis. A culture test looks to identify any bacteria present in the sample, which may indicate the cause of a urinary tract infection (UTI).

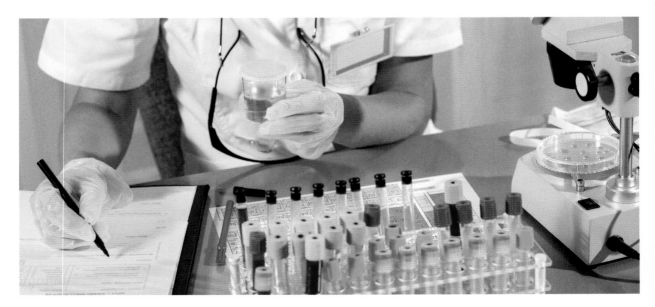

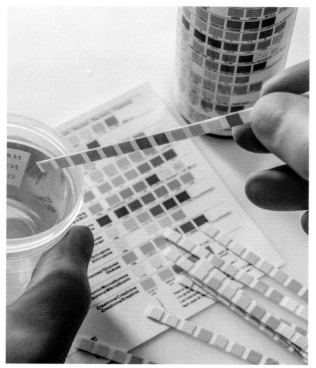

Dipstick test
A dipstick test uses a strip with coloured pads, which change colour when they react to the presence of a substance in the urine.

What is tested	Results
Leukocytes (white blood cells)	Usually suggestive of a urinary tract infection or contamination from vaginal discharge.
Nitrites	Nitrites are released by certain bacteria and their presence is suggestive of an infection.
Protein (proteinuria)	May represent damage to the kidney's filtration system due to diabetes, high blood pressure, kidney disease, or conditions such as myeloma.
pH (acidity/ alkalinity)	The pH of the urine can change as a result of your diet, kidney stones, or certain infections.
Ketones (ketonuria)	Ketones may be found in diabetic people with very high blood sugar (diabetic ketoacidosis), in those on low carbohydrate or starvation diets, and in urine that has been left stagnant.
Blood (haematuria)	Red blood cells in the urine may be the result of infection, stones, kidney disease, cancers, or contamination from menstrual blood.
Bilirubin and urobilinogen	May be seen in those with liver disease.
Specific gravity	This is a measure of how dilute or concentrated the urine is and depends on your hydration level.
Glucose/sugar (glucosuria)	Glucose is found in diabetic people's urine and this is a useful screening test for the condition.

Urine dipstick test

Urine can be tested rapidly using a multicoloured plastic strip that is dipped into your urine sample. Your healthcare professional will compare the strip to a colour scale, which correlates colour changes in the pads to possible abnormal findings in the urine, such as blood or glucose (see table, above right). Sometimes a machine may be used to analyse the pads. The level of changes in colour depend on how much of that substance is present, and this is graded using a plus sign.

Sending a sample to the lab

Urine can be examined under a microscope and cultured, where the bacteria are allowed to grow to identify which antibiotics may be used to treat infections. It usually takes around 72 hours for the results to be made available. The presence of abnormalities, such as red blood cells, white blood cells, casts, crystals, yeasts, and parasites, can be seen and counted using a microscope. Another test performed in the laboratory is to measure the amount of a protein called microalbumin. This measurement is used to calculate a score called ACR (albumin:creatinine ratio), which is used to monitor people with diabetes, hypertension, and kidney disease.

There are an estimated **150 million** cases of **urinary tract infections** globally **each year**

Testing kidney function

The kidneys act as filters, cleaning the blood and expelling waste via urine. Information on how well the kidneys are working can be obtained by tests done on a urine sample and on a blood sample.

URINE TEST FOR KIDNEY FUNCTION
The urine can be tested quickly and effectively by urinary dipstick analysis (see p.75) or by sending a urine sample to the laboratory (see p.75) for analysis.

What is tested
A dipstick test can identify infections, complications of diabetes, and damage to the kidneys, which may result in leakage of protein, ketones (a byproduct when fatty acids are broken down), or blood. A lab test of the level of a protein called microalbumin together with the amount of creatinine (a waste product of muscle) in the urine is used to calculate the albumin:creatinine ratio, or ACR. The urine for the ACR test is best collected as an early-morning sample. People with diabetes and those with raised blood pressure and protein in the urine should have an ACR done each year. A raised ACR (more than 3mg/mmol or 30 mg/g) is associated with an increased risk of chronic kidney disease and heart disease.

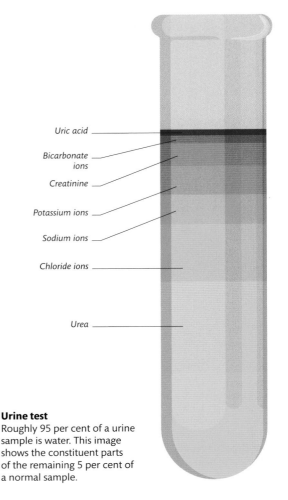

Uric acid

Bicarbonate ions

Creatinine

Potassium ions

Sodium ions

Chloride ions

Urea

Urine test
Roughly 95 per cent of a urine sample is water. This image shows the constituent parts of the remaining 5 per cent of a normal sample.

Microalbumin test
Healthy kidneys will retain necessary components of blood, such as the protein albumin. If there is kidney damage, albumin is one of the first proteins to leak out and be expelled in urine.

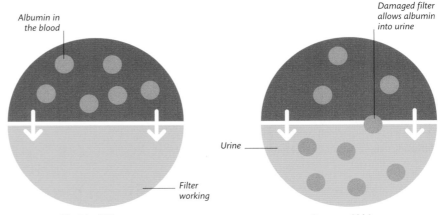

Albumin in the blood

Damaged filter allows albumin into urine

Urine

Filter working

Healthy kidney

Damaged kidney

BLOOD TEST FOR KIDNEY FUNCTION

A blood sample is taken in the usual way (see p.54) and sent to the lab for kidney function tests, also sometimes known as U&E (urea and electrolytes).

What the results mean

The blood is measured for the quantity of urea, creatinine, and electrolytes or salts, and the estimated glomerular filtration rate (eGFR) is calculated.

Urea and creatinine are both waste products passed into the urine via the kidneys, and if the organs are not working properly the levels in the blood of both are increased. They can rapidly increase and then lower again in normally healthy individuals following an episode of dehydration, stones, or severe infection, or due to certain medications. This is known as an acute kidney injury (AKI). The levels of salts or electrolytes can fluctuate due to kidney damage or conditions related to other organs.

The general function of the kidneys and how they do their job of filtering the blood can be determined by calculating the eGFR. This is calculated based on your age, sex, and ethnicity. The estimation can be affected by your build, dehydration, and amputation or muscle wasting. A normal eGFR has a value over 90ml/min/1.73m². If two tests are found to show eGFR below this level, over 90 days apart, this may indicate chronic kidney disease (CKD). Unlike AKI, CKD is a chronic or long-term condition that may progressively worsen.

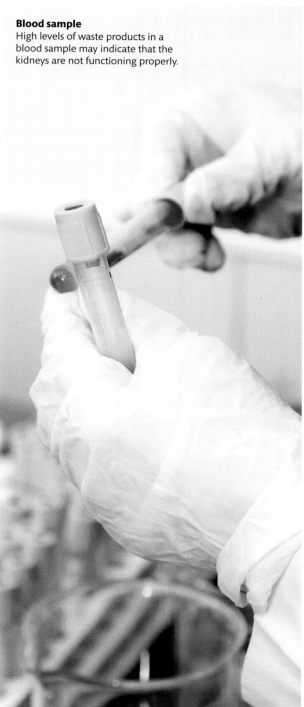

Blood sample
High levels of waste products in a blood sample may indicate that the kidneys are not functioning properly.

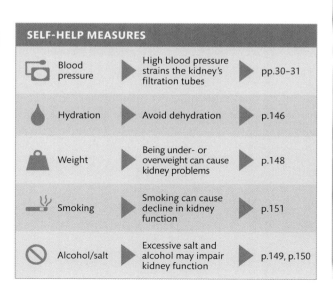

SELF-HELP MEASURES

Blood pressure	High blood pressure strains the kidney's filtration tubes	pp.30–31
Hydration	Avoid dehydration	p.146
Weight	Being under- or overweight can cause kidney problems	p.148
Smoking	Smoking can cause decline in kidney function	p.151
Alcohol/salt	Excessive salt and alcohol may impair kidney function	p.149, p.150

The male reproductive system

The male reproductive system comprises the penis and testes, the prostate gland, the passages and ducts connecting these parts, and the urethra. These organs and structures make and carry sperm, which fertilize a woman's eggs during sex.

Structures and functions

Sperm are made and stored in the testes. They travel through a system of passages and ducts to the penis, passing via the prostate gland, which adds liquid nutrients, creating semen. During sexual intercourse, the penis becomes erect, so that it can penetrate a woman's vagina, and semen exits the body via the urethra. The urethra also forms part of the urinary system, connecting to the bladder and enabling urine to leave the body.

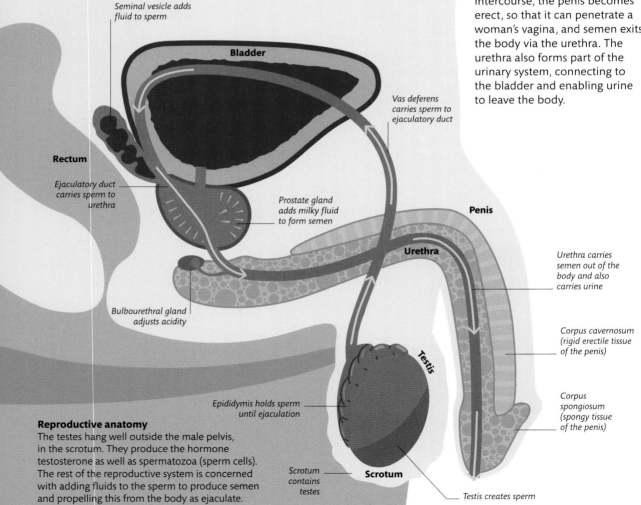

Seminal vesicle adds fluid to sperm

Bladder

Vas deferens carries sperm to ejaculatory duct

Rectum

Ejaculatory duct carries sperm to urethra

Prostate gland adds milky fluid to form semen

Penis

Urethra

Urethra carries semen out of the body and also carries urine

Bulbourethral gland adjusts acidity

Testis

Corpus cavernosum (rigid erectile tissue of the penis)

Corpus spongiosum (spongy tissue of the penis)

Epididymis holds sperm until ejaculation

Reproductive anatomy

The testes hang well outside the male pelvis, in the scrotum. They produce the hormone testosterone as well as spermatozoa (sperm cells). The rest of the reproductive system is concerned with adding fluids to the sperm to produce semen and propelling this from the body as ejaculate.

Scrotum contains testes

Scrotum

Testis creates sperm

Structure of the penis

The penis contains three columns of spongy tissue: the corpus spongiosum, holding the urethra, and two corpora cavernosa. During sexual arousal, extra blood is carried to the penis, making the corpora cavernosa (singular: corpus cavernosum) expand; this constricts the veins, so blood builds up in the penis, making it erect. After ejaculation, the pressure decreases and the blood drains away, so the penis becomes flaccid.

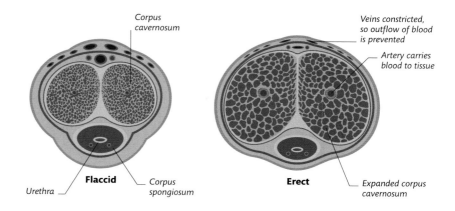

Corpus cavernosum

Veins constricted, so outflow of blood is prevented

Artery carries blood to tissue

Flaccid

Urethra

Corpus spongiosum

Erect

Expanded corpus cavernosum

The testes

Sperm cells are created inside the two testes, in tightly coiled tubes called seminiferous tubules. Here, they develop a head, containing the genetic material (DNA), and a tail, which helps them move. They then pass to the epididymis, where they become fully mature and mobile. Other specialized cells in the testes secrete testosterone, the male sex hormone.

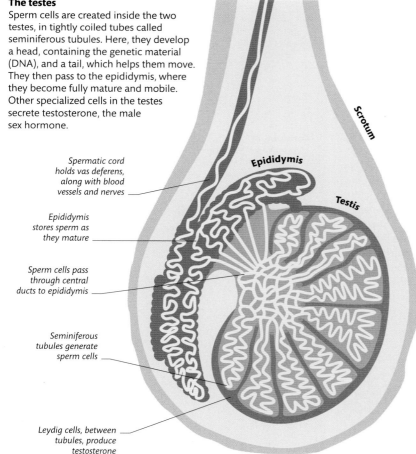

Spermatic cord holds vas deferens, along with blood vessels and nerves

Epididymis stores sperm as they mature

Sperm cells pass through central ducts to epididymis

Seminiferous tubules generate sperm cells

Leydig cells, between tubules, produce testosterone

Scrotum

Epididymis

Testis

MALE REPRODUCTIVE HEALTH CHECKS

The most common tests are carried out on samples of urine or blood, to detect sexually transmitted infections (STIs) or to screen for cancer. It is important to identify STIs promptly because they can be passed on to sexual partners, and they can affect fertility in a man or his partner. Men can be screened for signs of prostate cancer. To detect any early signs of testicular cancer, men should examine their own testes for lumps regularly.

A man can produce more than 500 billion sperm cells in his lifetime

Checking for infections

Men and women (see pp.88–89) can contract and spread sexually transmitted infections (STIs). They do this through unprotected vaginal, anal, or oral sex, or just close genital contact – with male or female partners. Some STIs can be transmitted via infected blood, saliva, or from mother to baby. STIs may produce no symptoms, so it is sensible to have an STI check before starting a sexual relationship, to reduce the risk of infecting others.

Blood tests

Some viral infections can be detected by blood tests. At the time of infection, HIV may cause a flu-like illness, but 1 in 5 people develop no symptoms. HIV is detected with a blood test for antibodies raised by the body against the virus. Antibodies can take 3 months to multiply sufficiently to give a positive result, so the best HIV tests look for antigens (traces of the virus itself) as well, which can be detected 4 weeks after infection.

If using "point of care" testing, at a sexual health clinic for instance, results can be produced from a pinprick blood sample on-site within a few minutes. In some clinics, you might be asked to provide saliva. A second test to confirm the results is strongly recommended.

Hepatitis C is also often asymptomatic. Blood tests look for antibodies, but in this case, antibodies can only show that the body has been exposed to the virus – it may since have fought the virus off. To confirm you are infected (and infectious), more precise tests are needed that detect the viral RNA (genetic material).

More than 1 million sexually transmitted infections are acquired every day worldwide

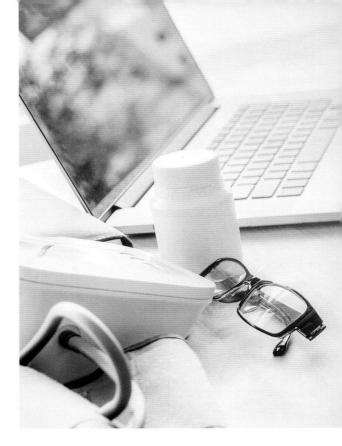

Consultation
If you suspect you have an STI, a clinician will ask you about your sexual history as part of the testing procedure. You might be asked when you last had sex, and if you used a condom.

Infection	Agent	Symptoms
HIV	Viral	
Hepatitis B	Viral	
Hepatitis C	Viral	
Genital warts	Viral	All of these infections can produce symptoms in some cases, but any of them can also be completely asymptomatic, particularly in the early stages
Genital herpes	Viral	
Syphilis	Bacterial	
Gonorrhoea	Bacterial	
Chlamydia	Bacterial	
Non-gonococcal urethritis	Bacterial	
Trichomoniasis	Protozoan parasite	
Pubic lice	Animal parasite	Visible lice (crabs)

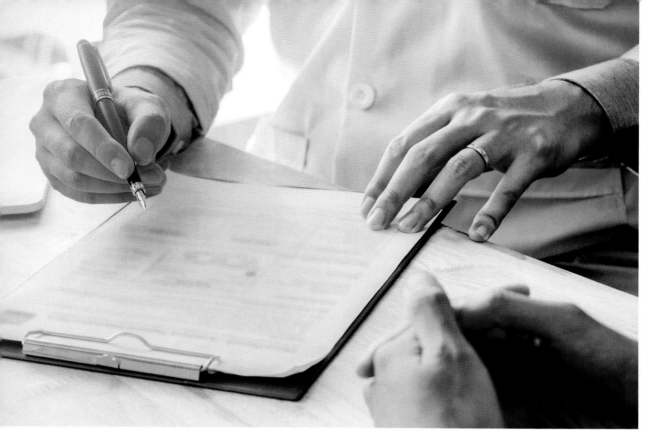

Urine tests and swabs

Bacterial infections, such as chlamydia and gonorrhoea, can be detected in urine or in swabs from the urethra. In the case of urine, you will be asked to wait for at least 2 hours since you last urinated before passing a urine sample. The first part of the urine stream should be caught in a sterile container. This is because, by the end of urination, vital telltale bacteria might have been washed away.

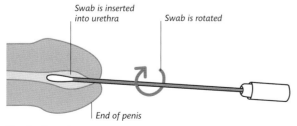

Swab is inserted into urethra

Swab is rotated

End of penis

Urethral swab test
The healthcare professional may want to take a swab. A small cotton-tipped swab is inserted directly into the urethra to collect any bacteria there. A swab can also be used to collect a specimen from your anus, throat, or eyes.

TESTING AT HOME

Home testing and home sampling HIV kits are available and legal in some countries. Most of them use a pinprick blood sample and/or a urine sample. You can sometimes do postal testing too.

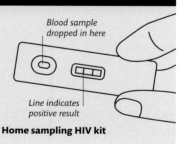

Blood sample dropped in here

Line indicates positive result

Home sampling HIV kit

SELF-HELP MEASURES

Vaccination	Discuss with your doctor having the hepatitis B vaccine	pp.144–45
Sex	Practise safer sex	pp.162–63

Checking the testicles

Caught early, testicular cancer is treatable and curable. If you start checking your testes in your teens, you will know what normal feels like, so you can spot early signs if they develop. You might feel a painless lump or heaviness in your testes or one of them might feel different from the other. Testicular cancer most commonly affects men aged 15 to 49.

Self checking

The best time to check your testes is after a warm bath. The heat allows the scrotum to relax and the testes to drop so it is easier to feel them. Try to do this once a month so you get familiar with how your testes feel.

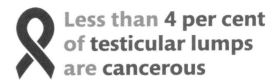
Less than 4 per cent of testicular lumps are cancerous

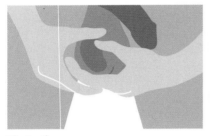

The testis
Examine one testis at a time. Roll it gently between your thumb and first two fingers. Feel for lumps or changes in the size, consistency, and shape. Check the other testis and make sure it feels similar.

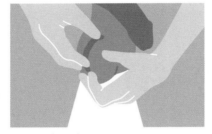

The epididymis
The epididymis sits at the back of the testis and feels a little squishy and rope-like. This is normal.

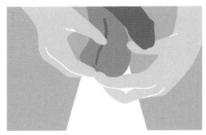

The vas deferens
The vas deferens feels like a firm, smooth, movable tube running behind each testicle. Run your thumb and forefinger along its length, in both testicles, feeling for lumps or tenderness.

What you might find

If you feel a lump it is unlikely to be cancerous, but you cannot decide this yourself, so seek medical advice. Most are caused by harmless conditions, such as an epididymal cyst or swollen veins around the testes called a varicocele. Your doctor will examine you and may shine a light through your scrotum to check if there is a build-up of fluid. You may then need an ultrasound scan of your testes, and possibly also blood tests, to determine if a lump is cancerous.

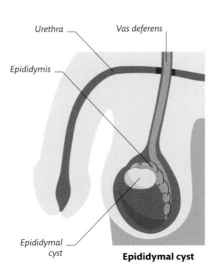

Urethra *Vas deferens*

Epididymis

Epididymal cyst

Epididymal cyst

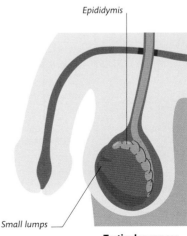

Epididymis

Small lumps

Testicular cancer

Checking the prostate

As you get older, your prostate tends to enlarge and can put pressure on your urethra. This may cause no symptoms or you might have difficulties passing urine. In many men, the enlargement is benign, although sometimes it may be due to prostate cancer.

Digital rectal examination
To undergo this examination, you will need to remove your underwear and lie on a couch on your left side. The doctor will ask you to bend your legs towards your chest.

The prostate gland

The prostate, a plum-sized gland that adds fluid to semen (see p.78), is present only in men. An enlarged prostate may make it hard to start or stop passing urine, it might make you go more often, or you might feel unable to empty your bladder completely. The enlargement may be harmless, but the chances of it being cancerous are greater if you are of Afro-Caribbean ethnicity or have a family history of prostate cancer or breast cancer.

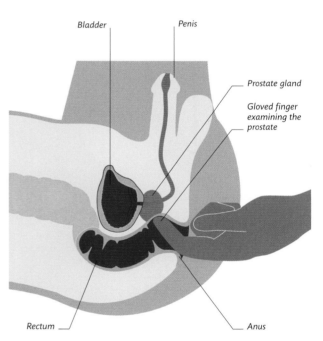

Bladder | Penis

Prostate gland

Gloved finger examining the prostate

Rectum | Anus

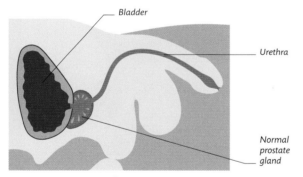

Bladder

Urethra

Normal prostate gland

Normal prostate

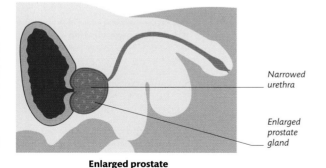

Narrowed urethra

Enlarged prostate gland

Enlarged prostate

Prostate enlargement
The urethra passes through the prostate gland, so if the prostate swells, it can compress the urethra, narrowing it and, in some cases, affecting urination.

Prostate tests

A diagnosis of prostate cancer is based on a series of tests, but the first step might be a digital rectal examination (DRE) or a blood test for prostate-specific antigen (PSA). During DRE, your doctor examines your prostate through the rectum. Using lubricating gel, they will insert a gloved finger. Your doctor will be able to feel if the prostate is enlarged or unusual in consistency.

The PSA test is not very specific. The PSA level can be raised if you have prostate cancer but also by non-cancerous causes such as age, benign enlargement of the prostate, or urinary tract infections. You may also have prostate cancer even if you have a normal PSA level. If your PSA is raised, you may be referred for an MRI (magnetic resonance imaging) scan of your prostate or a prostate biopsy (removal of a sample of prostate tissue for analysis).

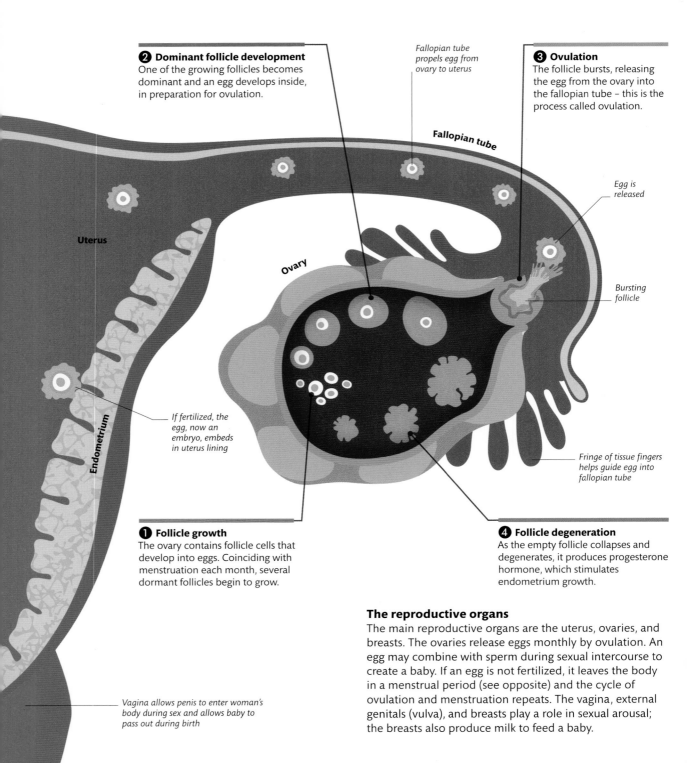

❷ Dominant follicle development
One of the growing follicles becomes dominant and an egg develops inside, in preparation for ovulation.

Fallopian tube propels egg from ovary to uterus

❸ Ovulation
The follicle bursts, releasing the egg from the ovary into the fallopian tube – this is the process called ovulation.

Fallopian tube

Egg is released

Uterus

Ovary

Bursting follicle

If fertilized, the egg, now an embryo, embeds in uterus lining

Endometrium

Fringe of tissue fingers helps guide egg into fallopian tube

❶ Follicle growth
The ovary contains follicle cells that develop into eggs. Coinciding with menstruation each month, several dormant follicles begin to grow.

❹ Follicle degeneration
As the empty follicle collapses and degenerates, it produces progesterone hormone, which stimulates endometrium growth.

The reproductive organs
The main reproductive organs are the uterus, ovaries, and breasts. The ovaries release eggs monthly by ovulation. An egg may combine with sperm during sexual intercourse to create a baby. If an egg is not fertilized, it leaves the body in a menstrual period (see opposite) and the cycle of ovulation and menstruation repeats. The vagina, external genitals (vulva), and breasts play a role in sexual arousal; the breasts also produce milk to feed a baby.

Vagina allows penis to enter woman's body during sex and allows baby to pass out during birth

The female reproductive system

The reproductive system in women includes the sex organs and the uterus (left), which holds a fetus (developing baby) during pregnancy. The system is controlled by hormones. Tests may be carried out to detect problems with either the body structures or the hormone levels.

The menstrual cycle

A woman's body goes through the menstrual cycle every month, when an egg is released (left) and the uterus lining thickens to receive it (below). The process is controlled by the hormones oestrogen and progesterone, produced in the ovaries, and follicle-stimulating hormone (FSH) and luteinizing hormone (LH), secreted by the pituitary gland. Menstruation continues from puberty until the menopause, when the ovaries stop responding to FSH and decrease their hormone production.

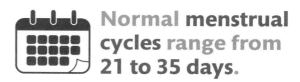

Normal menstrual cycles range from 21 to 35 days.

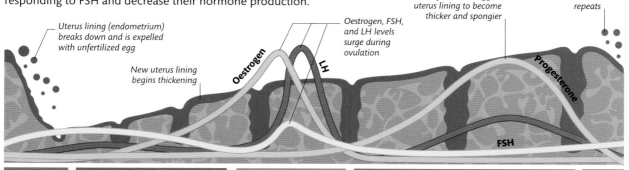

Uterus lining (endometrium) breaks down and is expelled with unfertilized egg

New uterus lining begins thickening

Oestrogen

LH

Oestrogen, FSH, and LH levels surge during ovulation

Progesterone triggers uterus lining to become thicker and spongier

Menstruation repeats

Progesterone

FSH

Menstruation   **Endometrium growth**   **Hormone surge**   **Further hormones**

Stages of the menstrual cycle

A menstrual cycle starts with a period, when an unfertilized egg is expelled from the body. Ovulation occurs at mid-cycle. If the egg is not fertilized, the uterus lining breaks down, repeating the process.

Breasts

Most of a woman's breast tissue consists of lobules – glands that produce milk during late pregnancy and after a birth. The milk passes along ducts to the nipple. The lobules are supported by fat and connective tissue.

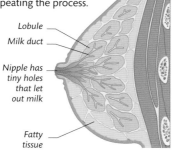

Lobule

Milk duct

Nipple has tiny holes that let out milk

Fatty tissue

FEMALE REPRODUCTIVE HEALTH TESTS

One of the most common tests for women is a urine test to detect pregnancy hormones. Other urine or blood tests may be carried out to identify hormonal disorders or sexually transmitted infections. Women may have regular screening with smear tests to detect cervical cancer, or mammograms to detect breast cancer. Other tests for diagnosing problems include blood tests to investigate causes of heavy or absent periods, imaging such as pelvic ultrasound, or viewing of the vagina, cervix, and uterus.

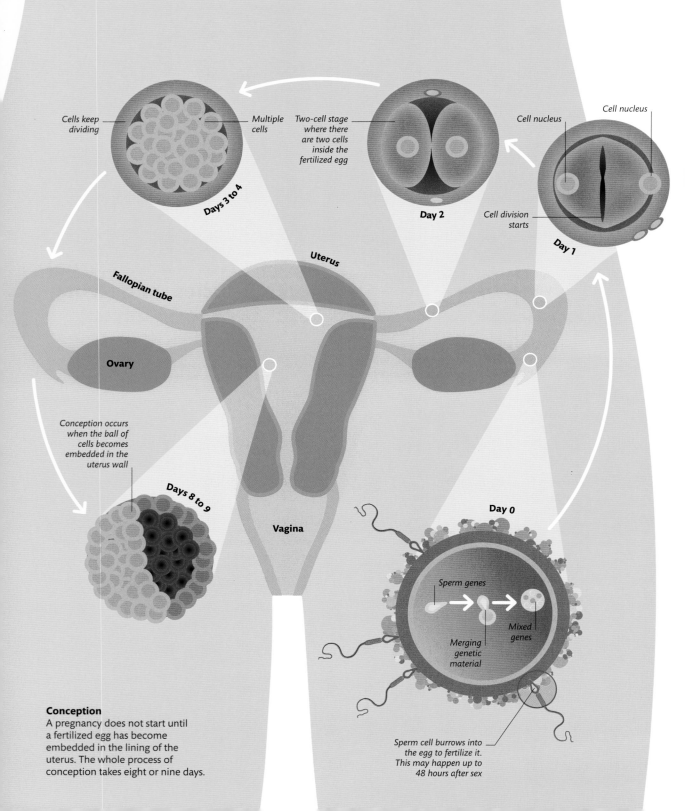

Cells keep dividing

Multiple cells

Two-cell stage where there are two cells inside the fertilized egg

Cell nucleus

Cell nucleus

Cell division starts

Days 3 to 4

Day 2

Day 1

Uterus

Fallopian tube

Ovary

Conception occurs when the ball of cells becomes embedded in the uterus wall

Days 8 to 9

Vagina

Day 0

Sperm genes

Merging genetic material

Mixed genes

Conception
A pregnancy does not start until a fertilized egg has become embedded in the lining of the uterus. The whole process of conception takes eight or nine days.

Sperm cell burrows into the egg to fertilize it. This may happen up to 48 hours after sex

Testing for pregnancy

A pregnancy test is a quick and reasonably accurate test to show if you are pregnant or not. The test is usually done using a urine sample and can be performed either at home or in the consulting room.

What the test involves

As soon as a woman falls pregnant, her body starts producing an increased amount of a hormone called human chorionic gonadotropin (hCG). Pregnancy tests detect the presence of hCG in either the urine or the blood.

The urine test involves either peeing onto a test strip, dipping the test strip into a small sample of urine, or using a small pipette to drop urine onto the strip. In each case there is a small chemical reaction if hCG is present and the strip will show this either by a colour change, a line appearing on the strip, or by indicating it digitally. Some newer tests can even tell you how many weeks pregnant you are.

The urine pregnancy test can show whether you are pregnant as soon as you have missed your period. This will be about two weeks since you actually conceived. However, there are some very sensitive tests that can be used as early as six days before a period is due.

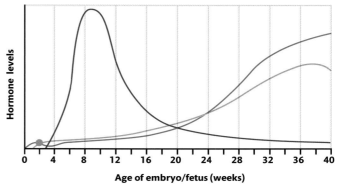

Age of embryo/fetus (weeks)

Pregnancy hormones
In the early stages of pregnancy, the production of human chorionic gonadotropin (hCG) increases sharply. Testing for this hormone is used to determine pregnancy.

KEY
— **Human chorionic gonadotropin (hCG)**
— **Oestrogen**
— **Progesterone**
● **Ovulation**

What the results mean

If the pregnancy test is positive, it usually means that you are pregnant. Rarely, however, the test can be positive although you are not pregnant. This might occur if the test is done soon after you have given birth or had a miscarriage or if you are taking certain medications. Likewise, the test can occasionally be negative although you are actually pregnant. This might occur if the test is done too early or the particular test kit is not very sensitive. If you think you are pregnant and the test is negative, it is a good idea to repeat the test about a week later or ask your doctor for an hCG test, which is more accurate.

When your pregnancy test is positive, you should arrange to see your doctor for ante-natal care. You should also discuss whether you should be taking any vitamins, such as folic acid. However, if you have abdominal pain or bleeding then you should see your doctor immediately as these may indicate a medical emergency.

HOME TEST

Home pregnancy tests are readily available from pharmacies, chemists, and supermarkets in many countries. They use a sample of your urine to detect hCG, but they may vary, so always follow the instructions. Results are available in a few minutes. The convenience of the test means it can be used as soon as you have missed your period. Some are sensitive enough to be done six days before your period is due, but none is 100 per cent accurate. Tests may be more accurate if an early morning sample is used, especially in very early pregnancy.

Result strip

Home test kit

Checking for infections

Gynaecological and sexually transmitted infections can be diagnosed by various tests. Before any tests are done, you will be asked about your gynaecological and sexual history and symptoms, such as abnormal vaginal discharge, itching, soreness, abdominal pain, or whether you are feeling unwell.

What to expect

There are three main types of test to check for infection; a blood test (see p.54), a urine test (see pp.74–75), and a vaginal swab. A swab is one of the most common tests you may have. The swab is a thin plastic stick with a cotton-wool tip. It is gently wiped across the area where there may be infection or discharge. In order to see the area inside the vagina, your doctor will use a small plastic or metal viewing instrument called a speculum. The end is coated with lubricating gel, then gently inserted into the vagina and the swab will be taken. However, you may be given a swab at the clinic so that you can take the sample yourself. Sometimes swabs are taken from sore places on the outside genital area and occasionally from the anus.

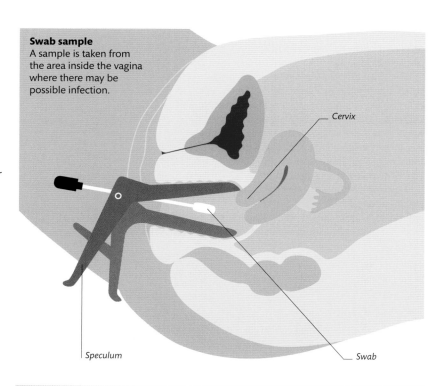

Swab sample
A sample is taken from the area inside the vagina where there may be possible infection.

Cervix

Speculum

Swab

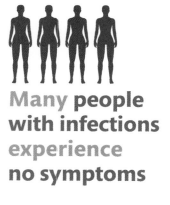

Many people with infections experience no symptoms

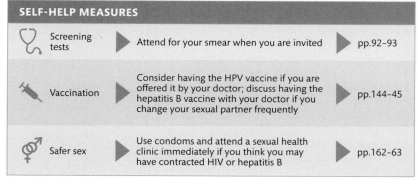

SELF-HELP MEASURES

	Screening tests	▶	Attend for your smear when you are invited	▶	pp.92–93
Vaccination	▶	Consider having the HPV vaccine if you are offered it by your doctor; discuss having the hepatitis B vaccine with your doctor if you change your sexual partner frequently	▶	pp.144–45
Safer sex	▶	Use condoms and attend a sexual health clinic immediately if you think you may have contracted HIV or hepatitis B	▶	pp.162–63

What the results mean

Any blood, urine, or swab samples are usually sent for testing in a laboratory. If the tests indicate that you have an infection, your doctor will recommend specific treatment appropriate for the infection, such as antibiotic tablets or cream.

TAKING A SWAB AT HOME

You may be given a swab kit by the clinic to take a sample yourself, or you can also buy home self-testing kits.

Step 1	Before taking the sample, wash your hands thoroughly with soap and water.
Step 2	Remove the swab from the packaging, ensuring that you do not touch the bud end. Hold the other end with your thumb and forefinger.
Step 3	You can sit or stand to take the swab. Put the tip of the swab stick about 2cm (¾ in) inside the vagina – approximately where you insert a tampon.
Step 4	Rotate the swab for 15–30 seconds.
Step 5	Place the swab into its container. You will need to label and date the sample before sending it off.
Step 6	Wash your hands with soap and water.

Swab held at top end

Cotton-wool tip

Container **Swab kit**

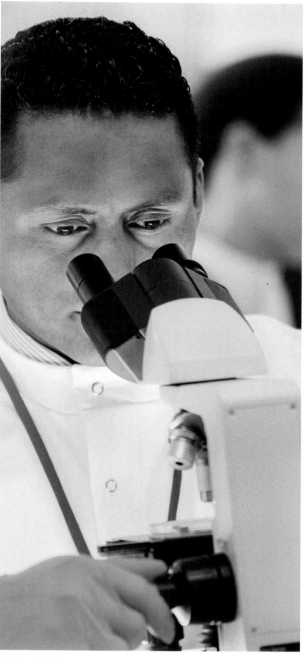

A closer look
Some infections are best diagnosed by using a urine or blood sample. Samples sent to the lab may be viewed under a microscope to look for abnormalities.

Pelvic examination

A pelvic or internal examination is an examination of your genital area and internal reproductive organs. It may be done if you have symptoms such as abnormal vaginal discharge, period problems, or lower abdominal pain.

What the test involves

You should always be asked if you would like a chaperone present for this type of examination. You will be required to remove your underwear and then lie on your back on the examination couch with your knees bent up and legs slightly apart or with your feet in stirrups. The doctor will wear disposable gloves for this examination and will first inspect the area around the outside of the vagina and then insert a speculum with gel on it gently into the vagina. The speculum is then opened slightly so that the inside of the vagina and the neck of the uterus can be seen. A cervical smear and swabs can be taken if necessary. Finally, the doctor will use two fingers to feel gently inside the vagina, with the other hand on your lower abdomen. Sometimes you may also be sent for an ultrasound scan. These tests may be slightly uncomfortable but should not be painful.

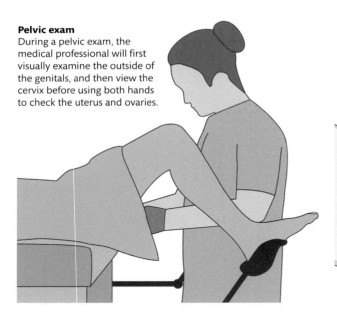

Pelvic exam
During a pelvic exam, the medical professional will first visually examine the outside of the genitals, and then view the cervix before using both hands to check the uterus and ovaries.

One hand will press down on the abdomen during the internal exam

Ovary

Uterus *Cervix*

Doctor will wear disposable gloves during the exam

What the results mean

These tests can show whether you have any abnormality in the genital region or cervix or whether you may have a vaginal or pelvic infection. The ultrasound scan can show if your uterus is enlarged or has a thickened lining or if you are pregnant. It can also check for cysts in the ovaries. Following these, your doctor may recommend further tests or treatment.

Colposcopy

This is an outpatient test to look at your cervix in detail to check for abnormal cells. It is done using a special microscope, called a colposcope, that resembles a pair of binoculars.

What the test involves

You may be sent for a colposcopy if your cervical screening test (see pp.92–93) has shown abnormal cells, if your cervix looks abnormal, or if you have symptoms, such as bleeding after intercourse. It should not be done during your period and you should avoid intercourse and using tampons or vaginal cream, gel, or tablets for two days before the test.

The test is similar to having a pelvic examination. The doctor will insert the speculum to get a clear view of the cervix. The colposcope is then used to look at your cervix although it does not touch or go inside you. A vinegar-like solution will be brushed onto the cervix, which reveals any areas where there are abnormal cells. This may sting a little but should not be painful. If there are any abnormal cells, the doctor can then take a small biopsy of this area and send it to the laboratory for analysis.

What the results mean

The test might show that your cervix is healthy and you will be advised to have regular smears. Sometimes the biopsy will show abnormal cells and this may need further tests or treatment.

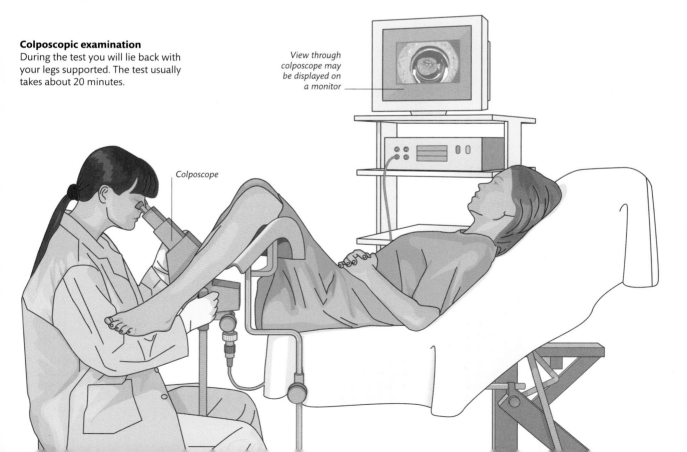

Colposcopic examination
During the test you will lie back with your legs supported. The test usually takes about 20 minutes.

View through colposcope may be displayed on a monitor

Colposcope

Checking for cervical cancer

A cervical, or Pap, smear is a test to checks whether or not the cells of the cervix are healthy. Cells are removed and analysed for either the presence of a virus, which can cause cancer, or for pre-cancerous cells, which can be treated before they can develop into cancer.

Why this test is important

A smear is a screening test to help prevent cancer. Cervical cancer is thought to be caused mainly by certain types of a sexually transmitted virus called human papillomavirus (HPV). Therefore women who have ever had any kind of sexual contact, regardless of when it was, should have regular smears. This includes lesbians and trans men who still have a cervix. You should also have smears even if you have had the HPV vaccine. However, if you have never had any sexual contact you may decide not to have this test.

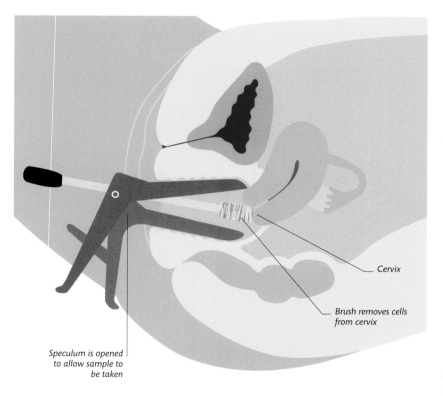

Globally, cervical cancer is the fourth most common cancer in women

Speculum is opened
to allow sample to
be taken

Cervix

Brush removes cells
from cervix

Cervical screening test

A smear, also sometimes called a cervical screening test, requires cells to be taken from the cervix. The vagina is held open with a speculum while the sample is taken. Cells are then examined for abnormalities.

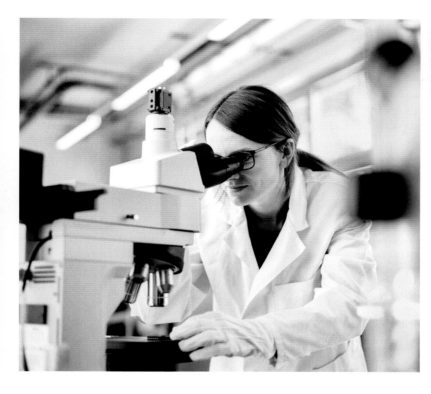

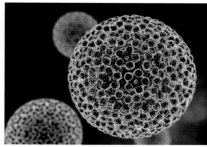

Cancer-causing virus
Certain strains of HPV are thought to be the cause of nearly all cases of cervical cancer. Screening for the virus is becoming an important way to determine the initial risk of someone developing cervical cancer.

Cytology
If a cancer-causing strain of HPV is found in the smear test, the individual cells are examined under a microscope for abnormalities. This is called cytology.

What the test involves

Initially you will be asked some questions regarding your periods and sexual history and you should be offered a chaperone. The test is very similar to having an internal pelvic examination (see p.90). The cervix is seen using a speculum, which may be lubricated with a small amount of gel. Cells from the cervix are removed, usually with a small brush. The cells are sent to the lab in a small pot containing a special liquid. Having the test may be slightly uncomfortable, although it should not be painful. It will also help if you can relax.

You should avoid having a smear during a period and should not have intercourse or use spermicidal cream or jelly for 24 hours beforehand.

What the results mean

You should receive your results in 2–4 weeks. Most people will have a negative (normal) result. A positive result may indicate either the presence of the HPV or abnormal cells seen on cytology. The nature of the cell changes found will determine whether you are followed up with another smear or referred for colposcopy (see p.91) to examine the cervix in more detail.

TABLE OF RESULTS

Result	What it means
Negative or normal	No action needed – you should have another routine smear in 3–5 years.
Inadequate	There were not enough cells in the sample and the test needs to be repeated. It does not mean anything is wrong.
Positive or abnormal	Cancer-causing strains of HPV were found to be present in the sample. The sample will then be checked for any abnormal cells and further tests or treatment will depend on whether or not any abnormalities are found.

Checking for breast cancer

Breast cancer is one of the most common forms of cancer worldwide and many countries have a screening programme that offers regular mammograms, usually after the age of 50 (or earlier if certain risk factors are present). Early detection increases survival rates, as the earlier the cancer is treated, the more effective the treatment will be.

BREAST AWARENESS
To pick up breast abnormalities as early as possible, a breast self-check should be done regularly. This could be once a month or after your period.

What the test involves
First, look at your breasts in a mirror. Start with your arms by your sides, then lift them up, and put your hands on your hips. Next, feel each breast, one at a time, using the hand opposite to the breast you are checking. This should be done when you are standing up and then when you are lying down, with the arm on the side you are examining lifted above your head. Use the flat part of your fingers and run your hand in a circular motion over all the breast tissue. Remember to check the breast going right up into your armpit and also going up to your collarbone. Gently squeeze around the nipple to check for any discharge or bleeding.

What to look for
Check for changes in the shape and contour of the skin and breasts, and any in the nipples. Examine the skin for changes such as puckering, dimpling, or any redness. And look for any breast lumps or swellings in the armpit. See your doctor immediately if you find any new changes or abnormalities. Remember that most lumps are not cancer, but it is always vital to get them checked by your doctor.

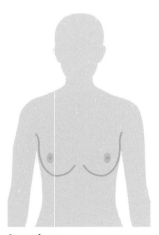

Arms down
Stand in front of a mirror with your arms at your sides and examine each breast. Look for any changes in shape, size, or symmetry.

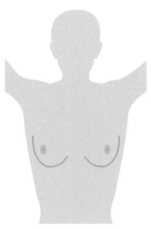

Arms raised
Raise your hands above your head and check for changes. Always look for swelling, lumps, or changes in the skin or nipple.

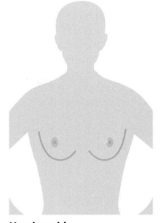

Hands on hips
Now, place your hands firmly on your hips. Again see if you notice any visible changes. Remember to check up to the armpit and the collarbone.

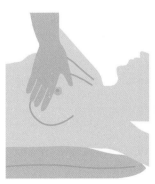

Lying down
Move your hand in small circles, pressing all around each breast, including the nipple and armpit. Feel for any changes, swelling, or lumps in the breast tissue.

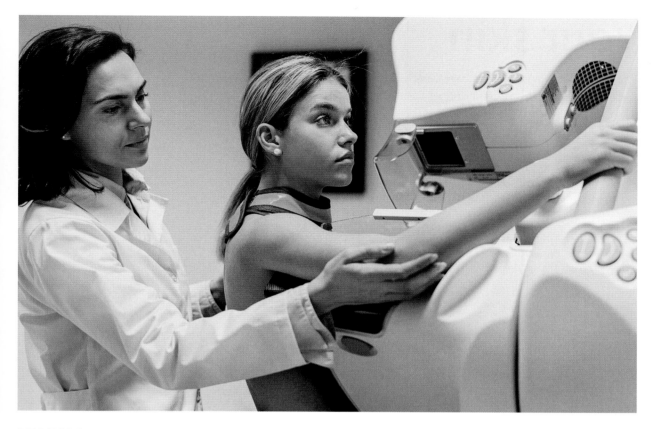

MAMMOGRAPHY

A mammogram is a low dose X-ray of your breasts that can show changes in your breast tissue, which may be breast cancer. This early detection of cancer can allow you to have treatment much sooner and will increase the chance of a cure.

What to expect

The mammogram takes about 10 minutes and it can pick up abnormalities even though your breasts can look and feel normal. You will first be required to remove your top clothes, including your bra. The X-ray is taken while you are standing up and each breast is X-rayed separately. The radiographer will stand you next to the machine and position your arm so that the whole breast can be seen. Your breast will then be placed on the machine's X-ray plate and a second plate will slowly be lowered onto the breast to gently squeeze it while the X-ray is being taken. This is often uncomfortable and occasionally painful, although this pressure only lasts for a few seconds. Each breast will usually be X-rayed from above and from the side.

Screening for cancer
A technician positions a patient's hand on the X-ray machine in order to ensure that she is aligned correctly for the mammogram to be taken.

What the results mean

In most cases the mammogram is normal, and you will then just be called back for a further routine screen in the future. If the mammogram result is unclear, you may be called back for a repeat test. If your mammogram shows any abnormalities, you will be called back for more tests. The radiologist will compare your latest mammogram to any others you have had in the past to see if the appearances are new or not.

If there are changes, you may have a breast examination, another mammogram, and an ultrasound scan. To rule out breast cancer, you may have a biopsy. A small sample is taken out with a needle and examined under the microscope to look for cancerous cells (see p.172).

Your skin

Your skin forms a vital barrier between the body and its surroundings. It helps protect deeper tissues, and also plays a key role in regulating body temperature.

The skin of an adult covers an area of about 1.5–2 sq m (16–21 sq ft)

Structure and function of skin

The skin consists of a thin outer layer called the epidermis and a thicker inner layer called the dermis. The epidermis contains the pigment melanin, which determines skin colour and helps shield against damage from sunlight. The dermis gives the skin strength and flexibility. Embedded in the dermis are sebaceous (oil-secreting) glands, sweat glands, hair follicles, and sensory nerve endings. Beneath the dermis is the fatty hypodermis, which provides insulation and also acts as an energy store.

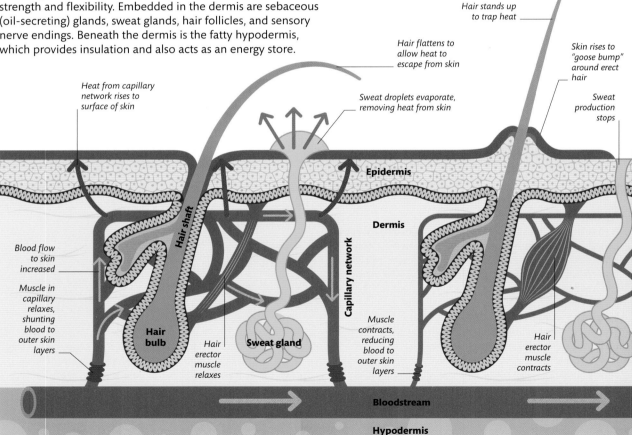

Hair stands up to trap heat

Skin rises to "goose bump" around erect hair

Hair flattens to allow heat to escape from skin

Sweat production stops

Heat from capillary network rises to surface of skin

Sweat droplets evaporate, removing heat from skin

Blood flow to skin increased

Muscle in capillary relaxes, shunting blood to outer skin layers

Hair shaft

Hair bulb

Hair erector muscle relaxes

Sweat gland

Capillary network

Muscle contracts, reducing blood to outer skin layers

Hair erector muscle contracts

Epidermis

Dermis

Bloodstream

Hypodermis

Hot-weather skin

When the body is hot, capillaries in the skin widen to increase heat loss from the skin's surface. The skin also produces sweat, which evaporates and takes heat away.

Cold-weather skin

When the body is cold, skin capillaries narrow to conserve body heat. Tiny muscles at the base of hair follicles contract, pulling body hairs upright to trap warm air near the skin.

CHECKING THE SKIN

Your skin reflects your general health and can reveal signs of a range of conditions. Checking the skin can therefore be a valuable health indicator. Changes in the skin may be caused by a disorder of the skin itself, such as skin cancer or a fungal infection, or may indicate a more general disease involving other body systems. Conditions affecting the skin often look different in dark skin and light skin.

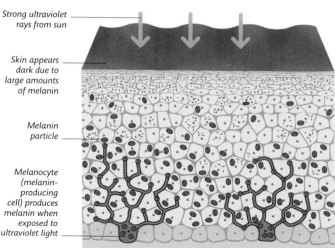

Strong ultraviolet rays from sun

Skin appears dark due to large amounts of melanin

Melanin particle

Melanocyte (melanin-producing cell) produces melanin when exposed to ultraviolet light

Dark skin
Dark skin contains large amounts of melanin, a pigment that helps to protect against ultraviolet rays in sunlight, which can trigger skin cancer. Vitamin D is made in skin exposed to ultraviolet light, and people with dark skin are at risk of deficiency if they receive too little sunlight.

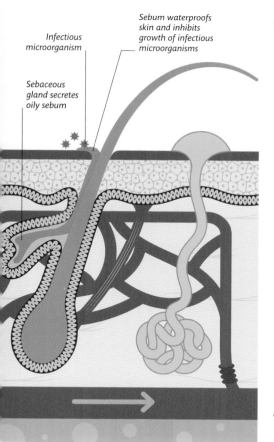

Infectious microorganism

Sebum waterproofs skin and inhibits growth of infectious microorganisms

Sebaceous gland secretes oily sebum

Defensive barrier
The epidermis is a tough, waterproof layer whose dead surface cells are constantly replaced by new cells from beneath. Sebum reduces water loss from the skin surface and protects against infection.

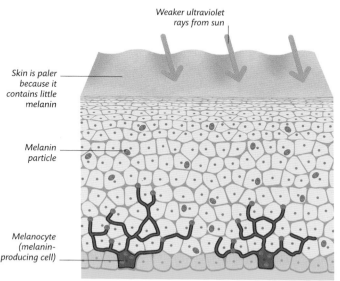

Weaker ultraviolet rays from sun

Skin is paler because it contains little melanin

Melanin particle

Melanocyte (melanin-producing cell)

Pale skin
Pale skin contains small amounts of melanin but this is usually sufficient to protect against the weaker ultraviolet rays from the sun outside equatorial regions. However, people with pale skin are more at risk of skin cancer if they are exposed to a lot of sunlight.

Checking your skin

Regularly checking your skin can help to detect any problems early, when they are more easily treatable. Most skin complaints are minor but some, notably melanoma, are potentially serious and require prompt medical evaluation. Some skin problems may also indicate an underlying disorder that may require medical intervention.

Skin examination

It is important to check your skin regularly for any abnormalities, especially any new moles or changes to existing ones, which may indicate melanoma skin cancer (see below). Check your entire skin in a well-lit area. Use a mirror or ask somebody else to check areas you cannot see yourself. It is useful to photograph the size, position, and appearance of moles. If you spot anything unusual, you should consult a doctor, who will perform a detailed examination, including inspecting the skin with a dermoscope and possibly taking whole-body images to map all your moles.

Signs of possible skin cancer

Features of moles that may indicate melanoma include asymmetrical shape, irregular border, uneven colour, size over 6mm (¼ in) and any change in appearance. You should also look out for any other unusual lump, sore, or blemish that grows, darkens, hurts, itches, bleeds, or does not heal within about four weeks.

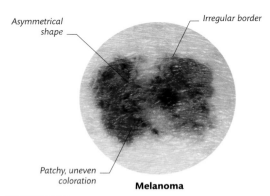

Asymmetrical shape

Irregular border

Patchy, uneven coloration

Melanoma

Dermoscopy

Dermoscopy involves a detailed inspection of the skin with a magnifying instrument (a dermoscope). The dermoscope may be connected to a digital imager, which enables the images to be enhanced to aid accurate identification of abnormalities.

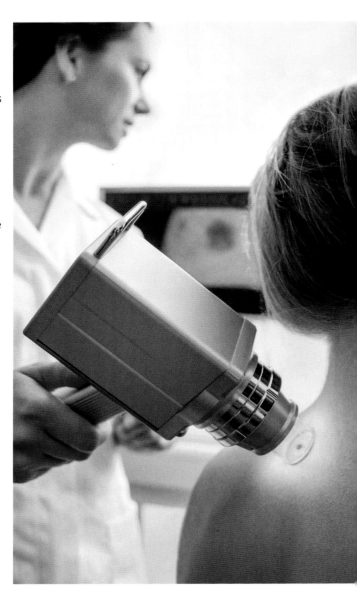

Common skin problems

Although skin problems are common, they are not usually serious and often clear up without treatment or with simple self-help measures, such as using an over-the-counter preparation for a mild fungal infection (athlete's foot, for example). The table (right) outlines typical features of some common problems. To confirm what the problem is, you should consult a doctor, especially if it persists, worsens, or recurs. The doctor will also be able to advise you about suitable treatment.

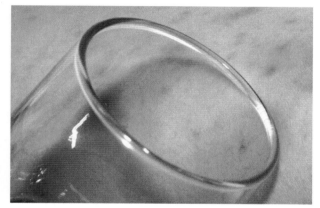

Glass test for meningitis
A type of bacteria that can cause potentially life-threatening meningitis can also cause a rash. The rash usually starts as tiny purplish spots. It does not fade if you press a clear glass against the skin. In dark skin, the rash may be easier to see on the palate or in the eyes. Meningitis is a medical emergency.

PROBLEM	TYPICAL FEATURES
Psoriasis	Thickened patches with silvery scales; an autoimmune disorder
Seborrhoeic dermatitis	Scaly, itchy patches on scalp (dandruff) and face
Athlete's foot	Itchy, sore, cracked skin between toes due to fungal infection
Ringworm	Itchy, ring-shaped patches due to fungal infection
Urticaria	Rash of itchy, raised lumps or patches due to allergic reaction
Skin tag	Soft lump that hangs from the skin
Blister	Fluid-filled swelling just under skin surface
Cold sores	Painful cluster of tiny blisters near edge of lips due to a virus
Sunburn	Painful, red, hot areas on skin exposed to sun
Warts and verrucas	Firm, rough growths; verrucas are warts that flatten into the soles of the feet
Corns and calluses	Thickened areas on hands or feet in areas of pressure or friction
Bruise	Dark, discoloured area from bleeding under the skin due to injury, a blood disorder, or some medications
Insect bites	Small, itchy lumps that may have a tiny central bite-hole
Boil or abscess	Painful, pus-filled spot or lump due to bacteria
Acne	Pimples, spots, and greasy skin on face due to bacteria
Folliculitis	Pus-filled pimples around hair follicles due to bacteria
Cyst	Rounded, fluid-filled lump
Eczema	Dry, itchy patches on skin

SELF-HELP MEASURES

Diet	Eat a well-balanced diet	pp.146–47
Smoking	Quit smoking	pp.150–51
Ultraviolet light	Avoid excessive exposure to sunlight and other sources of ultraviolet light; use sunblock with an SPF of 30 when outdoors	pp.158–59

How the eyes work

The eyes take in light and focus it, producing sharp images. Their internal structures adjust automatically to control the focal length and the level of light entering the eye for optimum vision.

The retina contains 120–150 million rod cells and 6–7 million cone cells

Structure of the eye

Structures at the front of the eye focus light on to light-receptive cells in the retina, deep inside the eyeball. Electrical signals from these cells pass along the optic nerve to the brain, which interprets the signals as images. Signals from both eyes are combined to give us depth perception. Muscles around the eyeball point the eye in different directions. The coloured part of the eye, the iris, controls the amount of light entering the pupil, so we can see in bright or dim light.

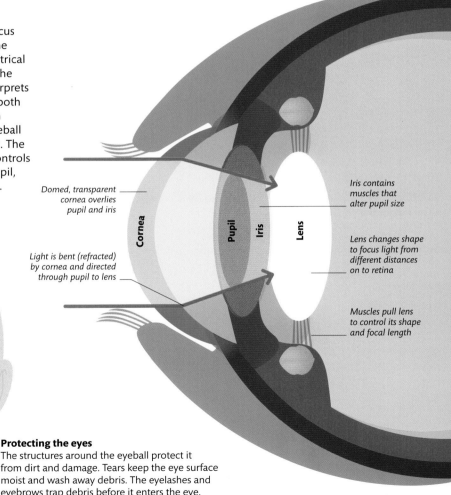

Domed, transparent cornea overlies pupil and iris

Light is bent (refracted) by cornea and directed through pupil to lens

Cornea

Pupil

Iris

Lens

Iris contains muscles that alter pupil size

Lens changes shape to focus light from different distances on to retina

Muscles pull lens to control its shape and focal length

Tear gland produces tears

Upper eyelid sweeps down to spread tears

Tears drain through tear duct

Excess tears overflow if eye is irritated or when we cry

Protecting the eyes

The structures around the eyeball protect it from dirt and damage. Tears keep the eye surface moist and wash away debris. The eyelashes and eyebrows trap debris before it enters the eye. The eyelids cover the eyes to protect them; they also spread tears across the eye by blinking.

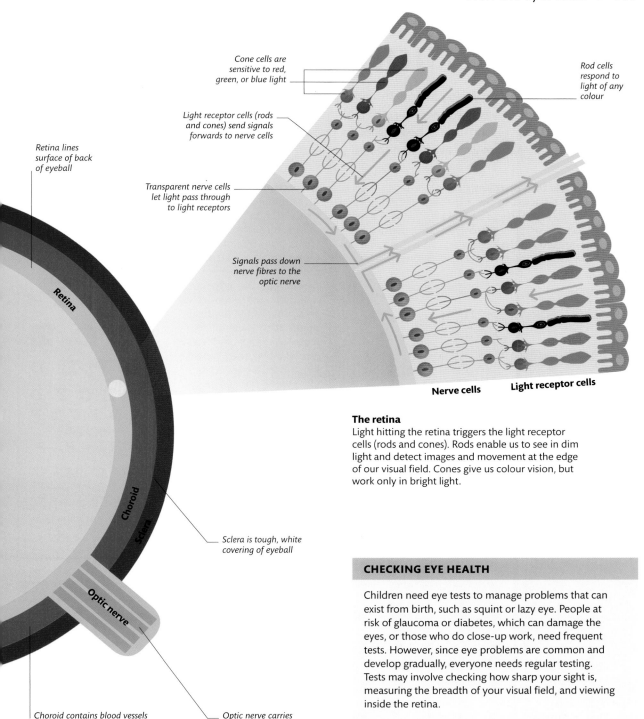

Cone cells are sensitive to red, green, or blue light

Rod cells respond to light of any colour

Light receptor cells (rods and cones) send signals forwards to nerve cells

Transparent nerve cells let light pass through to light receptors

Retina lines surface of back of eyeball

Signals pass down nerve fibres to the optic nerve

Nerve cells   **Light receptor cells**

Retina

Choroid

Sclera

Optic nerve

Sclera is tough, white covering of eyeball

Choroid contains blood vessels that supply retina and sclera

Optic nerve carries signals to brain

The retina
Light hitting the retina triggers the light receptor cells (rods and cones). Rods enable us to see in dim light and detect images and movement at the edge of our visual field. Cones give us colour vision, but work only in bright light.

CHECKING EYE HEALTH

Children need eye tests to manage problems that can exist from birth, such as squint or lazy eye. People at risk of glaucoma or diabetes, which can damage the eyes, or those who do close-up work, need frequent tests. However, since eye problems are common and develop gradually, everyone needs regular testing. Tests may involve checking how sharp your sight is, measuring the breadth of your visual field, and viewing inside the retina.

Testing vision

One of the main aims of an examination by an optometrist (healthcare specialist trained to examine the eyes) is to check for vision disorders – most commonly refractive, or focusing, errors that can be adjusted by prescribing corrective lenses. As eyesight changes with age, vision should be tested regularly.

Potential refraction problems

Light is bent, or refracted, by the cornea and the lens to focus an image on the retina. Focus can be affected by the length of the eyeball and shape of the cornea (astigmatism, see p.104). Age-related lens hardening also causes gradual loss of the ability to focus on close-up images (presbyopia).

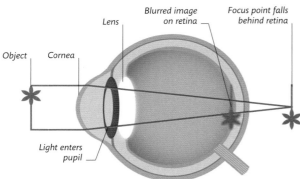

Object | Cornea | Lens | Blurred image on retina | Focus point falls behind retina | Light enters pupil

Long-sightedness

Difficulty seeing nearby (and to a lesser extent, distant) objects – hypermetropia – occurs if the eyeball is too short, but can be corrected with plus-powered (convex) lenses.

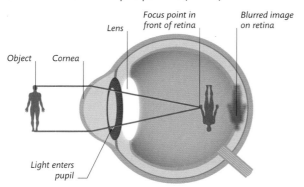

Object | Cornea | Lens | Focus point in front of retina | Blurred image on retina | Light enters pupil

Short-sightedness

Difficulty in seeing distant objects clearly – myopia – can occur if the eyeball is slightly too long, but can be corrected with minus-powered (concave) lenses.

Refraction testing

An optometrist will test your vision by asking you to look through a series of lenses using a phoropter (opposite) or a trial frame to find out whether you have a refractive error. If one is found, the lenses will be adjusted until the right prescription is identified. Distance refraction is always assessed first, then if extra lens power is needed for close work, this can be added to your prescription.

Snellen chart

To test visual acuity, you may be asked to read lines of letters of gradually decreasing size on a screen or chart, named after the Dutch ophthalmologist who designed it. Each eye will be assessed separately.

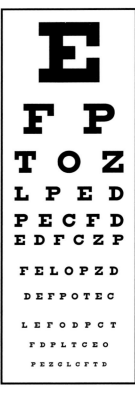

ONLINE VISION TESTS

A number of websites now offer rudimentary online eye tests. Depending on the site, there is a range of options, from visual acuity and contrast and colour vision tests, to assessment of the curvature of the cornea (astigmatism) and even field of vision (see p.108). They are useful as they can indicate whether your sight has changed, but should not be considered as a substitute for a check-up with an optometrist, as this will include a comprehensive eye-health examination.

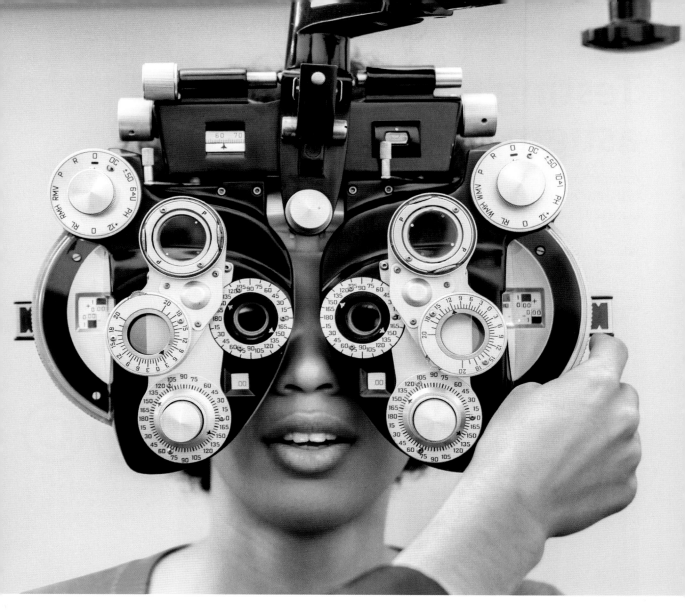

Assessment with a phoropter
This is a device, used instead of a trial frame, which holds different lenses that can be dropped in front of each eye. Some units are controlled manually, others via a computer.

It is a **myth** that wearing reading glasses for **presbyopia** weakens eye muscles

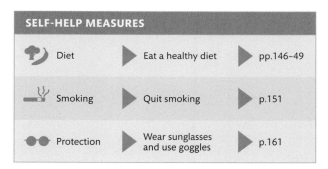

SELF-HELP MEASURES			
Diet	▶	Eat a healthy diet	▶ pp.146–49
Smoking	▶	Quit smoking	▶ p.151
Protection	▶	Wear sunglasses and use goggles	▶ p.161

Testing for astigmatism

Astigmatism is an irregular curvature of the cornea or the lens of the eye. It can cause light to be focused in more than one place within the eye, which can result in a blurred image.

33% of the population has astigmatism in one or both eyes

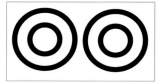

When is it tested?
Astigmatism can cause blurring of distance and near vision, in addition to focusing errors that accompany short-sightedness, long-sightedness, or presbyopia. The greater the difference in the curvature from the norm, the more difficult it is to focus. Your optometrist will check for astigmatism as part of the vision test (see p.102–103). Using a phoropter or a trial frame, they will present a series of lenses and ask you to look at circular targets (see right), then state when they appear clear and round.

What do the results mean?
Astigmatism does not go away. If it is mild, you may have no symptoms and require no treatment. If it is significant enough to cause blurred vision or eyestrain then it will require correction with glasses, contact lenses, or even laser surgery. The level of correction needed can be added to your prescription (see p.102).

If you wear contact lenses, the degree of astigmatism can also have a bearing on the type of contact lenses you can wear. Your optometrist may also need to take an exact measurement of the shape of the front of the cornea as well as the amount and alignment of the astigmatism, using a keratometer, or ophthalmometer (see below).

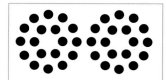

Focusing the circles
Your optometrist will either show you a pair of concentric circles (right) or circular patterns of dots (left).

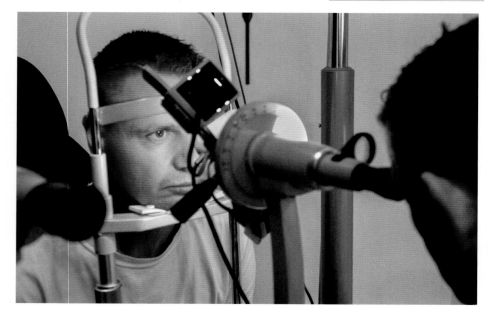

A keratometer in use
With your chin and forehead supported, the optometrist will shine a target onto the cornea. By observing its reflection in the keratometer eyepiece they can measure the surface curvature.

Colour vision test

People with colour vision deficiencies have difficulty identifying some colours or distinguishing between certain colours – typically red and green, and more rarely, blue and yellow – and will generally see fewer colours than people without them.

How colour vision is assessed

Most colour vision defects are inherited, and the need for testing will be identified when an optometrist takes a family history. It is recommended that all boys are screened, but a girl need only be tested if her mother or her male relatives are colour deficient, or if she appears to have difficulty recognizing certain colours.

The most commonly used colour vision test is the Ishihara test, named after the Japanese ophthalmologist who invented it, which is especially good for identifying red/green colour deficiencies. The test comprises 38 colour plates, including one control card, most of which have coloured numbers hidden within a pattern of different coloured dots. You will be shown the cards and asked to identify the numbers you can see. Another widely used test is the Farnsworth D-15 test, in which you will be asked to arrange 15 coloured discs in sequence.

What the results indicate

People with a hereditary deficiency do not have a disease and the condition does not change. Contrary to popular belief, those affected are not "colour blind" – it is very rare for a person to be unable to see any colours at all. The deficiency may be slight, moderate, or severe and may have an impact on potential career choices – tinted lenses can help in some cases. Some colour vision defects can develop later in life, but they are likely to be associated with drugs, disease, or toxins (from excessive drinking and smoking, for example). Acquired defects are usually worse in one eye than the other and more often associated with a blue/yellow defect; they may improve, but can worsen too.

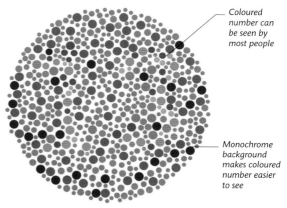

Coloured number can be seen by most people

Monochrome background makes coloured number easier to see

Introductory, control plate

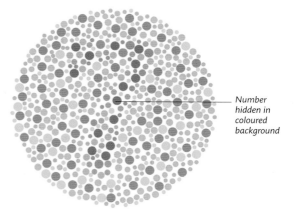

Number hidden in coloured background

Screening and classification plate

1 in 12 men and only 1 in 200 women have colour vision problems

Examples of Ishihara plates
The control plate is shown so you understand what is required in the test. Plates with coloured dots are used to indicate the type and level of colour deficiency.

Checking your eye health

As well as assessing your eyes for refractive errors, your optometrist will routinely check both the front and inside of your eyes. The check-up can reveal signs of eye-related health issues, from cataracts (lens clouding) to age-related macular degeneration; it can also indicate general physical conditions such as diabetes.

Examining the front of the eye

Your optometrist will begin by checking all the structures at the front of your eyes, from the eyelids and lashes to the body of the eye (see p.100), using a slit lamp. The lamp focuses a narrow beam of light onto the eye, enabling them to examine the eye through a microscope. The light is normally white, but green or blue light may be used; if it is the latter, then yellow dye will be instilled in your eye first.

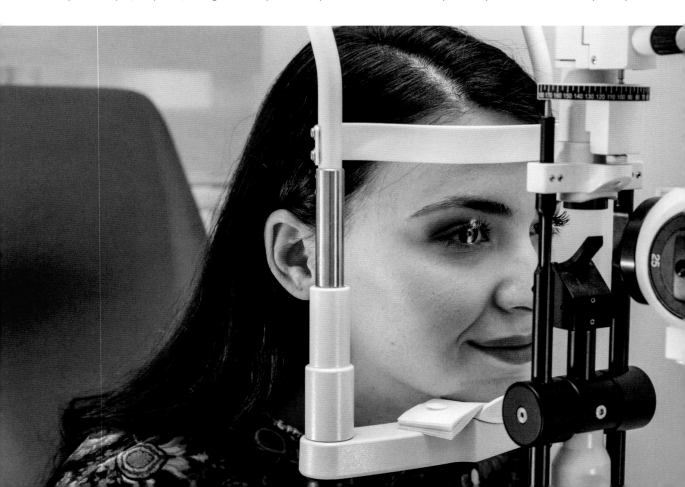

RETINAL PHOTOGRAPHY

A photographic image of the back of the eye (the fundus) provides a visual record of the health of your eyes and is a useful way to monitor any change in their appearance. Eyedrops may be needed to dilate the pupil sufficiently, and you will sit in front of the camera with your chin and forehead supported in a frame.

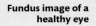

Fundus image of a healthy eye

Examining the inside of the eye

Using a handheld ophthalmoscope or a slit lamp, your optometrist will shine a light directly into each eye to examine the internal structures: lens, light-sensitive retina (including the macula), retinal blood vessels, the head of the optic nerve, and the vitreous humour that fills the eye. It may be necessary to instil drops to dilate the pupils. This is painless, but you may need to wear sunglasses for an hour or two afterwards and your vision may be blurred, so you will be advised not to drive.

An estimated 80% of all vision impairment worldwide is considered avoidable

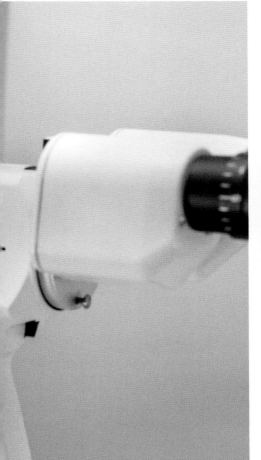

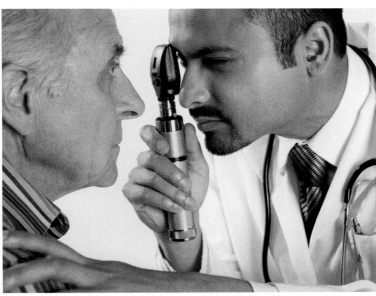

Ophthalmoscope examination

As the light is directed into your eye, you will be asked to look straight ahead, then right and left, and up and down, while the optometrist scans inside the eye.

Slit-lamp examination

You will need to place your chin on a rest and your forehead against a strap. The optometrist will direct a beam of light onto the front of each eye while looking through the eyepiece of the microscope.

Testing visual field

Also known as perimetry, this test assesses the extent, or perimeter, of your visual field. This is done routinely to determine whether you have a blind spot, or more frequently if you are at a high risk of glaucoma.

What to expect in the test

A confrontation test may be performed initially. Your optometrist will sit 1 m (3 ft) in front of you and ask you to look directly into their eye or at the tip of their nose. They will then wave their finger or an object at the edge of your visual field and ask you to indicate when you can see it. While this is not sensitive enough for fine assessment, it shows any major defects. An accurate assessment can be performed with automated perimetry testing, which "maps" your field of vision. You will sit at the machine while a set of lights flashes at the edge of your line of sight.

Understanding your results

If a defect is identified it is important that its size and position are analysed. You will need to be monitored more closely to check for any change. Your optometrist may refer you to an ophthalmologist to identify the possible cause.

Loss of peripheral vision severely affects ability to drive safely

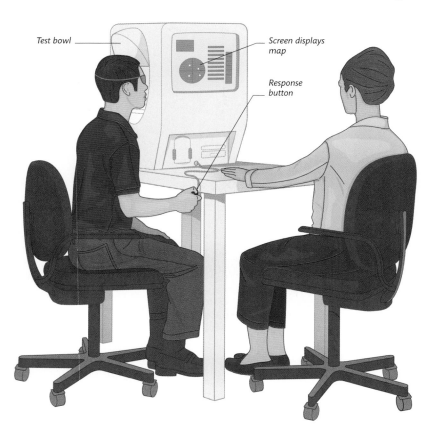

Test bowl

Screen displays map

Response button

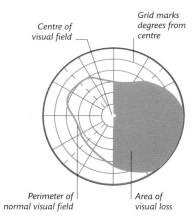

Centre of visual field

Grid marks degrees from centre

Perimeter of normal visual field

Area of visual loss

Visual field map

The perimetry machine tracks the position of the lights you do not see, and in doing so creates a "map" that shows the area of visual loss.

Automated perimetry test

If you wear glasses, the eye being tested will have your lens prescription placed in front of it; the other one will be covered. You will be asked to focus on the centre of the test bowl and press a response button each time you see a light flashing.

Measuring eye pressure

Your optometrist will routinely measure your internal eye (intraocular) pressure to determine whether you are at risk of developing glaucoma, a condition in which the optic nerve can be damaged by an abnormal build-up of pressure (ocular hypertension).

How is pressure measured?

Your eye is filled with a clear fluid that washes around inside it, passes through the pupil, and drains out through the "angle" between the cornea and the iris. The drainage channels can become blocked, leading to a build-up of pressure within the eyeball. Your eye pressure can be measured with a table-mounted or handheld non-contact tonometer, placed 1–2 cm ($^1/_2$–$^3/_4$ in) in front of your eye. This emits a painless puff of air at the cornea. It will make you blink, but by then the reading has already been taken.

Non-contact tonometry

This device measures the speed at which the cornea is flattened when a puff of air from the tonometer is directed at it, then gives an estimated reading of the intraocular pressure.

Tonometer nozzle

Air bounces off surface of cornea to give pressure reading

Fluid pressure in eye

Retina

Pupil

Lens

Cornea

Optic nerve

Direction of air from tonometer

Iris

What do the results indicate?

If your intraocular pressure is repeatedly raised, or is much higher in one eye than the other, a more precise measurement using applanation tonometry will be recommended. You may also be referred to an ophthalmologist for further tests and a more detailed examination before a full diagnosis can be made.

Glaucoma can lead to permanent loss of peripheral vision and even total blindness

APPLANATION TONOMETRY

Also known as contact tonometry, this is a very precise measurement in which a small tonometer probe is gently placed on the front of the cornea. Before the procedure, anaesthetic drops and dye will be put in your eyes. During the test, which takes a few seconds, the optometrist will observe the flattening of the cornea and take an exact reading of the intraocular pressure in each eye.

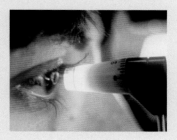

Tonometer in use

How the ears work

Our ears have two very important functions. The most obvious one is hearing, a process that involves the whole ear. A less familiar function is enabling balance, which is done by certain structures in the innermost part of the ear.

Structures of the ear

The ear has three main parts called the outer, middle, and inner ear. In the outer ear, the pinna (visible part) directs sound waves down the ear canal to the eardrum. The eardrum vibrates; this causes ossicles (tiny bones) in the middle ear to move, transmitting the vibrations to the inner ear. Here, the vibrations are converted to electrical signals that are sent to the brain, which interprets them as sounds. Also in the inner ear are structures that register our movements and orientation relative to gravity, to maintain our balance.

Your ears never stop hearing sounds, even when you are asleep 🎵

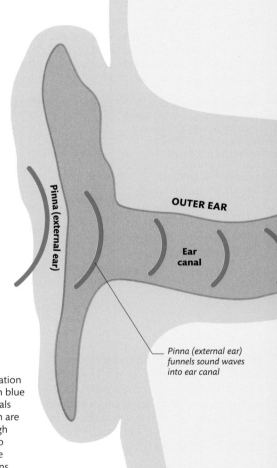

Pinna (external ear)

OUTER EAR

Ear canal

Pinna (external ear) funnels sound waves into ear canal

EAR TESTS

Most ear tests involve hearing. Babies and children are tested so that deafness can be picked up as early as possible. Adults may be tested for age-related hearing loss or to identify temporary problems such as earwax build-up or infection. Tests may involve examining your ear canal and eardrum and assessing your ability to hear sounds. Balance tests may involve the doctor moving your head and body to investigate problems that may be making you feel sick or unsteady on your feet.

Hearing pathway

The route of sound information through the ear is shown in blue in this illustration. The signals begin as sound waves, then are passed as vibrations through the eardrum and ossicles to a fluid-filled organ called the cochlea. Here, the vibrations are converted into electrical signals, which are passed along the auditory nerve to the brain.

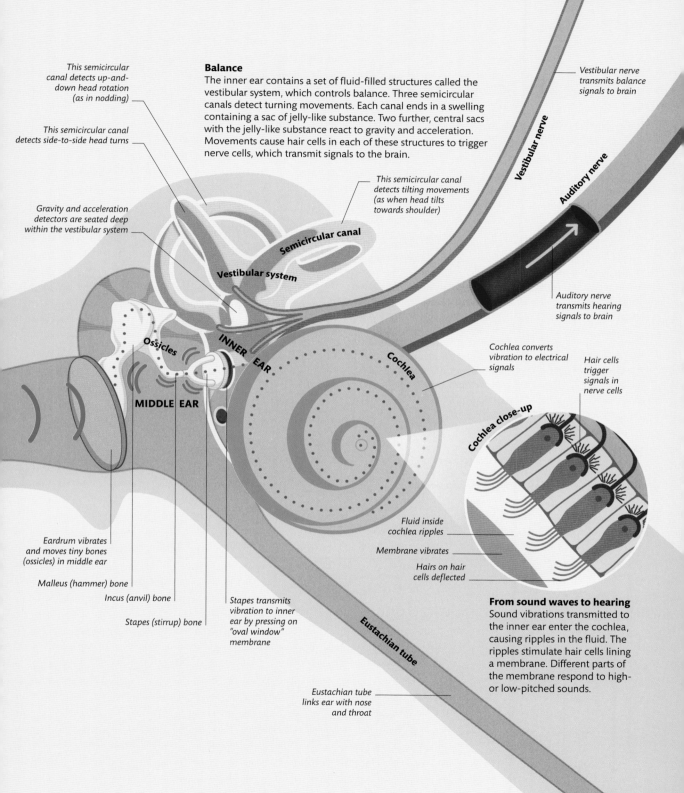

Balance

The inner ear contains a set of fluid-filled structures called the vestibular system, which controls balance. Three semicircular canals detect turning movements. Each canal ends in a swelling containing a sac of jelly-like substance. Two further, central sacs with the jelly-like substance react to gravity and acceleration. Movements cause hair cells in each of these structures to trigger nerve cells, which transmit signals to the brain.

This semicircular canal detects up-and-down head rotation (as in nodding)

This semicircular canal detects side-to-side head turns

Gravity and acceleration detectors are seated deep within the vestibular system

This semicircular canal detects tilting movements (as when head tilts towards shoulder)

Semicircular canal

Vestibular system

INNER EAR

Ossicles

MIDDLE EAR

Vestibular nerve

Vestibular nerve transmits balance signals to brain

Auditory nerve

Auditory nerve transmits hearing signals to brain

Cochlea

Cochlea converts vibration to electrical signals

Hair cells trigger signals in nerve cells

Cochlea close-up

Fluid inside cochlea ripples

Membrane vibrates

Hairs on hair cells deflected

Eardrum vibrates and moves tiny bones (ossicles) in middle ear

Malleus (hammer) bone

Incus (anvil) bone

Stapes (stirrup) bone

Stapes transmits vibration to inner ear by pressing on "oval window" membrane

Eustachian tube

Eustachian tube links ear with nose and throat

From sound waves to hearing

Sound vibrations transmitted to the inner ear enter the cochlea, causing ripples in the fluid. The ripples stimulate hair cells lining a membrane. Different parts of the membrane respond to high- or low-pitched sounds.

Testing your hearing

Untreated hearing loss has been linked with increasing the chances of developing dementia, a decrease in cognitive function, and also has possible links with depression. For these reasons, it is important to have your hearing checked throughout your lifespan.

Audiometry

Pure-tone audiometry is a test designed to measure the quietest sounds that you can hear. During the test you will listen to pure tones (sounds at a single, precise frequency, or pitch) at different volumes and frequencies. You listen through headphones and press a button each time you hear a sound. The results show the quietest sounds you can hear at each frequency and are plotted on a graph called an audiogram, with red circles for the right ear and blue crosses for the left. The graph shows a measure of hearing level against frequency. Any points that are heard at 20 decibels (dB) or quieter are considered to be within the normal range. The lower down the graph the points are plotted, the worse the hearing is.

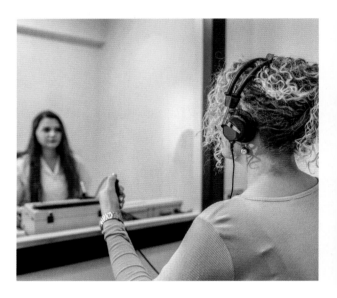

What the test involves

Audiometry is ideally carried out in a soundproof booth to isolate you from ambient noise. You press a button whenever you hear a sound in the headphones.

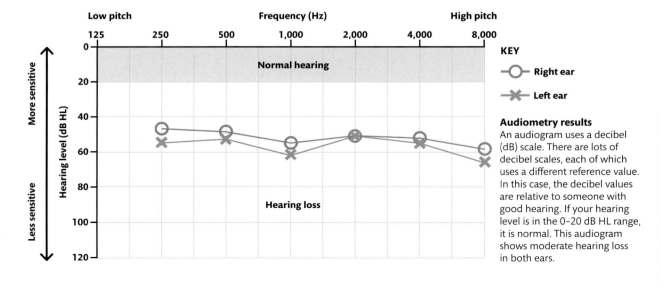

KEY

—O— Right ear

—✕— Left ear

Audiometry results

An audiogram uses a decibel (dB) scale. There are lots of decibel scales, each of which uses a different reference value. In this case, the decibel values are relative to someone with good hearing. If your hearing level is in the 0–20 dB HL range, it is normal. This audiogram shows moderate hearing loss in both ears.

Speech perception test

Pure tones, as used in audiometry (left), are rarely encountered in our day-to-day lives. The chart below shows the loudness and frequency of sounds as we commonly experience them, with speech sounds in yellow. Speech testing gives information that is more relevant to daily listening experiences. It is similar to pure-tone audiometry, but you will listen to words rather than sounds. It is a useful test to perform when considering hearing-aid provision, as it measures your ability to hear and interpret speech, and hearing aids are designed to improve the way you do this.

Noise at 100 dB can damage hearing in 15 minutes

The speech banana

The range of speech sounds we experience resembles a banana shape when plotted on a frequency-loudness chart. Extreme low- and high-frequency speech sounds tend to be fainter, but within normal hearing range. Listeners with even mild hearing loss, however, fail to hear these components of speech.

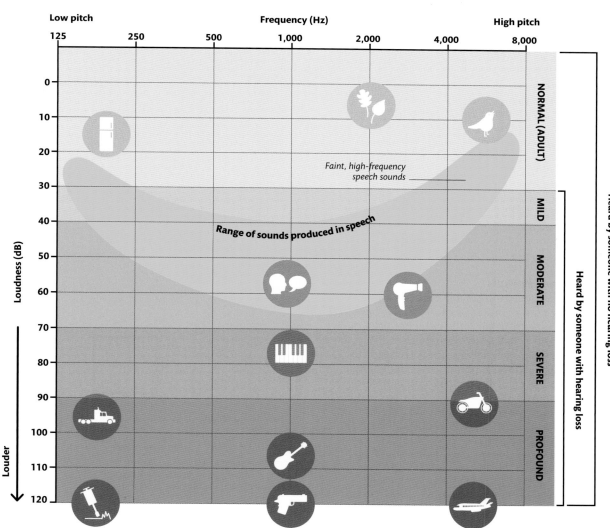

Tympanometry

Tympanometry is an examination used to test the condition of the middle ear and the mobility of the eardrum (tympanic membrane). It can help diagnose disorders that can lead to hearing loss, especially in children. The test measures the movement of your eardrum in response to changes in pressure.

What to expect
Tympanometry is a test to find out how effectively the middle ear transmits sound to the inner ear. When sound hits the eardrum, some is sent through the middle ear to the inner ear, while the rest is reflected from the eardrum. If the eardrum is functioning properly, it will be flexible and there will be little reflected sound; the admittance (also called compliance) of the ear is said to be high.

To begin the test, the audiology professional looks into your ear with an otoscope to check that there is nothing obstructing the ear canal. A tympanometer probe is then placed into the ear canal. The device emits a tone; it may feel slightly uncomfortable and you will hear some loud sounds as the device takes measurements. The probe changes the air pressure in your ear to move the eardrum back and forth, causing sensations similar to those you might feel during takeoff and landing on a plane. The test takes a few minutes.

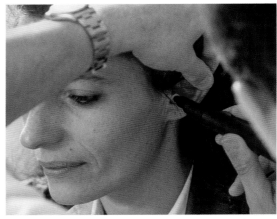

Tympanometer probe
The probe of a tympanometer has a soft rubber tip. The pressure of the rubber tip against the ear canal wall forms an airtight seal.

Interpreting the results
The graph produced, called a tympanogram, helps the audiology professional decide whether you have normal middle-ear function. If the test is normal, it means that there is no fluid in the middle ear, the eardrum moves normally, there is normal pressure in the middle ear, and there is normal movement of the ossicles (small bones) of the middle ear that conduct sound to the inner ear.

The most common reason for an abnormal tympanogram is fluid in the middle ear, but other common causes are perforation of the eardrum, earwax blocking the eardrum, lack of mobility or other problems with the ossicles of the middle ear, or a problem with the Eustachian tube, which links the nose and throat with the middle ear. If abnormal results are obtained, you may be referred to an ear, nose, and throat doctor for a medical opinion.

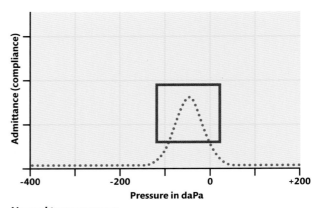

Normal tympanogram
The axes of a tympanogram show admittance (compliance) plotted vertically, while the pressure is plotted horizontally in decapascals (daPa). A peak in admittance in the box on the chart shows normal middle ear function.

Inside the ear canal

The tympanometer probe has three components – a loudspeaker that delivers a tone, a pump that varies the pressure in the ear canal, and a microphone that measures the sound reflected from the eardrum. The sound measurement is recalculated as admittance (also called compliance), which is a measure of how much sound is passed on, based on how much is reflected.

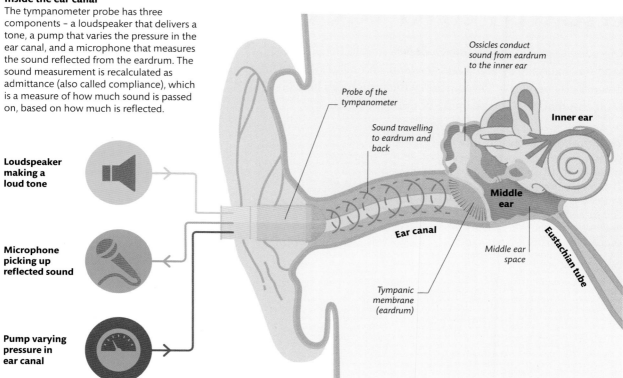

Loudspeaker making a loud tone

Microphone picking up reflected sound

Pump varying pressure in ear canal

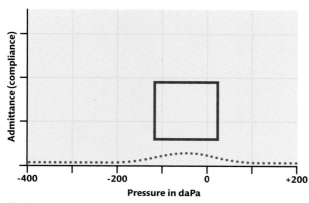

Flat tympanogram

A flat graph, or one with reduced admittance (compliance), suggests fluid in the middle ear or a perforated eardrum. Tympanometry also measures the volume of the ear canal, and if this figure is high and the graph is flat, then a perforated eardrum is likely.

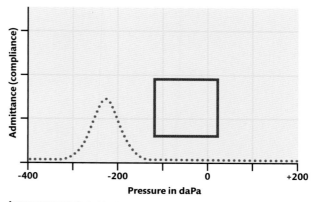

Low-pressure tympanogram

If there is normal admittance (compliance) at reduced pressure, this suggests middle ear congestion or Eustachian tube dysfunction (since the Eustachian tube is responsible for equalizing pressure in the ear and draining fluid from the middle ear).

Mouth and teeth

Digestion begins in the mouth. Our teeth start to break down food mechanically by biting and chewing, and saliva starts to break down food chemically. Proper care of the mouth can help prevent problems that could cause decay or even loss of teeth.

The structures of the mouth

When we take a bite of food, facial muscles move our jaws so our teeth can bite and chew to break down the food. The tongue moves food around so that saliva can get into it. Saliva is a fluid produced by three pairs of glands in the cheeks and under the tongue; it contains an enzyme that begins the breakdown of some food molecules. These actions reduce the food to a soft ball for swallowing.

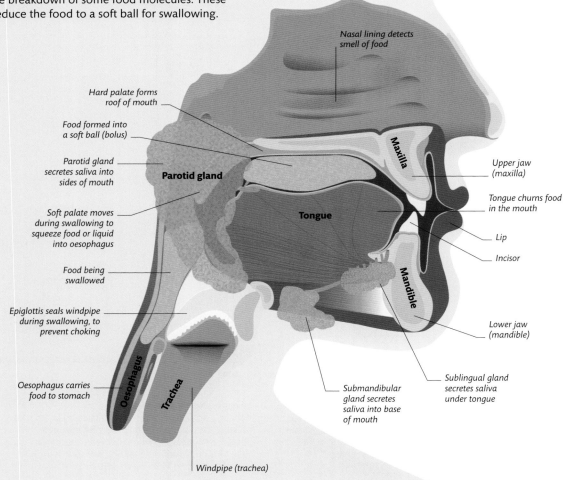

Nasal lining detects smell of food

Hard palate forms roof of mouth

Food formed into a soft ball (bolus)

Parotid gland secretes saliva into sides of mouth

Parotid gland

Soft palate moves during swallowing to squeeze food or liquid into oesophagus

Food being swallowed

Epiglottis seals windpipe during swallowing, to prevent choking

Oesophagus carries food to stomach

Maxilla

Upper jaw (maxilla)

Tongue

Tongue churns food in the mouth

Lip

Incisor

Mandible

Lower jaw (mandible)

Sublingual gland secretes saliva under tongue

Submandibular gland secretes saliva into base of mouth

Oesophagus

Trachea

Windpipe (trachea)

Tooth enamel

Teeth are covered by enamel, which is the hardest substance in the body, but it readily dissolves in acid, exposing the underlying parts of the tooth to bacteria and infection. Acid can come from some foods, juices, and fizzy drinks, or from bacterial plaque, which breaks down sugar to form lactic acid. If the entire thickness of enamel dissolves, it allows infection to rot the softer dentine beneath. Cavities can form as the weakened enamel collapses.

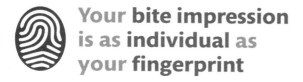

Your **bite impression** is as **individual** as your **fingerprint**

CHECKING ORAL HEALTH

Brushing your teeth every day can prevent problems such as a build-up of plaque, which can lead to tooth decay, or gum disease, which could expose the roots of your teeth to infection. You also need regular dental checks every 1–2 years. The dentist will examine your teeth and gums and remove any hardened plaque. You may be offered a scale and polish to clean your teeth, or an X-ray to assess problems such as hidden tooth decay or impacted teeth. The dentist can also advise you on diet and oral health. If you are nervous about visiting dentists, let them know before your appointment, and they will take care to put you at your ease.

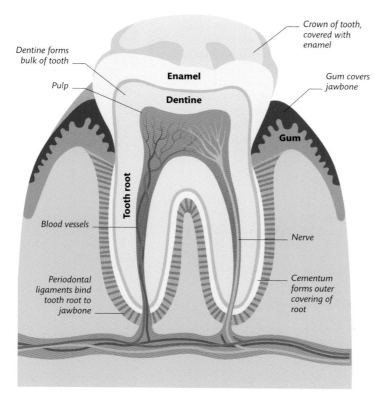

Dentine forms bulk of tooth
Pulp
Enamel
Dentine
Crown of tooth, covered with enamel
Gum covers jawbone
Gum
Tooth root
Blood vessels
Nerve
Periodontal ligaments bind tooth root to jawbone
Cementum forms outer covering of root

Structure of a tooth

Teeth are fixed into the jawbones by long roots. The crown (visible part) has a tough coating of enamel. Beneath this is hard material called dentine, and in the middle of the tooth is soft pulp. The gums form a seal around the bases of the teeth to keep out bacteria.

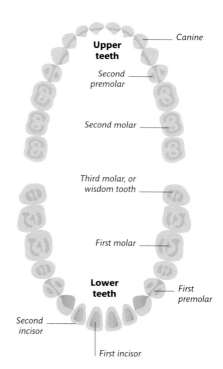

Canine
Upper teeth
Second premolar
Second molar
Third molar, or wisdom tooth
First molar
Lower teeth
First premolar
Second incisor
First incisor

Biting and chewing

A full set of teeth comprises four types, each doing a specific job. At the front of the mouth, incisors bite food into pieces, while canine teeth grip and tear. Further back, inside the cheeks, premolars and molars crush food into a paste.

Dental check-up

Regular visits to the dentist should form an integral part of your health monitoring. Tooth cavities and gum disease are preventable and your dentist can not only help you keep your teeth and gums healthy, but also identify signs of decay early.

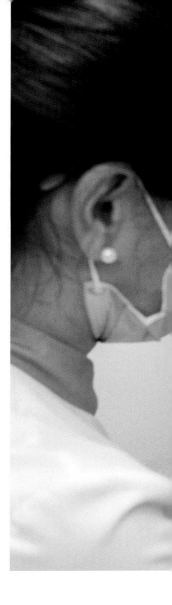

What to expect at a dental check-up

Your dentist will first ask about your general health and lifestyle habits, such as whether or not you eat a healthy diet, smoke, or are prone to clenching your teeth. They will also want to know if you are on any medication and whether you have had any known gum or tooth problems.

Your dentist will start by examining the underside of your jaw and neck, then look at, listen to, and feel the joints where the jawbone meets the skull for signs of deviation or noises that could indicate jaw problems. They will count your teeth and check each one, making a note of: the condition; existing fillings or crowns; signs of decay; and the extent of plaque and tartar buildup. They will also assess the health of the gums, your tongue, and soft tissues in your mouth.

An X-ray may be taken either in the form of a small plate that is placed in your mouth, then processed on a film or digitally, or using a larger machine that moves around your head. The latter examines the top and bottom jaws and shows not only the teeth, but also sinuses and nerve canals. Some dentists recommend repeat X-rays every few years.

Understanding the results

Depending on the findings, your dentist will discuss any potential treatment and/ or advise you when you should have your next check-up. Plaque can cause tartar build-up on your teeth, which leads to tooth decay and gum disease. Your dentist may clean the teeth to remove plaque and tartar or refer you to a hygienist. Signs of tooth decay may require further treatment. You may be referred to a specialist if the gum disease is severe or abnormalities are detected.

During the check-up
You will be given goggles to protect your eyes and a bib to protect your clothes. While your dentist examines the teeth and gums, a dental nurse will remove moisture that accumulates.

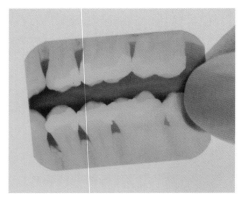

Use of X-rays in dental health
X-rays may be used to aid diagnosis of localized tooth decay, bone loss, infection, or impacted teeth not otherwise visible to the naked eye.

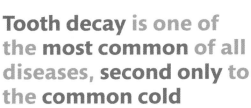

Tooth decay is one of the **most common** of all diseases, **second only to** the **common cold**

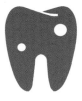

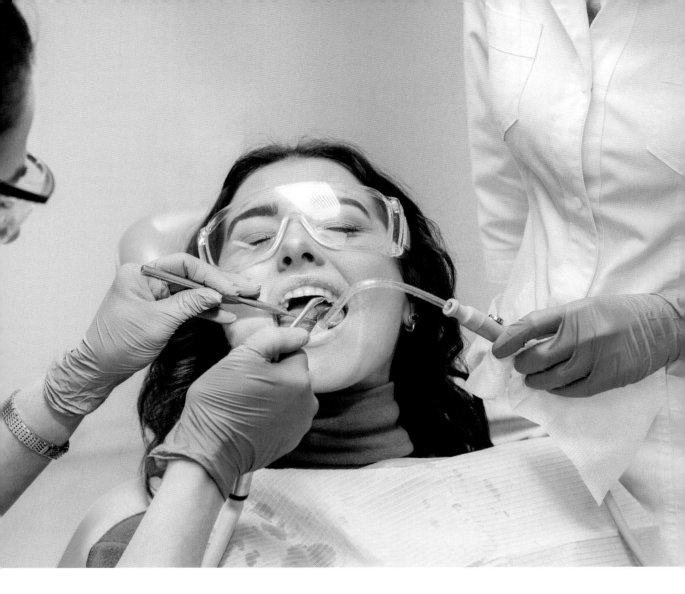

SELF-MONITORING

Check your mouth regularly and make an appointment to
see the dentist before your scheduled check-up if you notice:

- Toothache and/or increased sensitivity to hot or cold food
  or drinks.
- Facial swelling.
- Bleeding gums.
- Ulcers that will not heal or any unusual red or white
  patches that cannot be explained.

SELF-HELP MEASURES

Diet	Maintain a healthy diet	pp.146–49
Oral health	Clean teeth daily; avoid sugary foods	p.146
Alcohol and tobacco	Limit alcohol intake and do not smoke or chew tobacco	pp.150–51

Your skeleton

Our skeletal system is the framework that supports the body, protects our organs and other body structures, and enables us to move. It is formed from bone and connective tissues. There are 206 bones in all, linked together by a system of joints.

Bones and joints
Bones are living tissues, which form light but strong structures. Many bones have connective tissue called cartilage at their ends, and this reduces friction during movement, or connects certain bones (such as the ribs and sternum, or breastplate). Joints are the structures that connect one bone to another. The joints in the skull and pelvis are fused together, but most other joints allow movement; the bones in these joints are held together by tough, fibrous connective tissues called ligaments.

Spine structure
The spine consists of 33 vertebrae. These support the head, neck, ribcage, and lower back, and form part of the pelvis. The neck and back vertebrae allow bending and twisting. Ligaments hold the vertebrae together, while tough, springy cartilage discs between them act as shock absorbers during movement.

We have around **300 bones** when we are **born**, but some of these **fuse together as we grow**

Inside a joint
In movable joints, the bones are connected by ligaments. The bone ends are covered with a layer of tough cartilage, so they can move smoothly against each other. They are sealed in a joint capsule, filled with fluid (synovial fluid) that lubricates the bone ends.

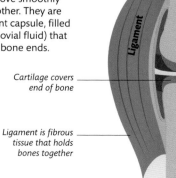

Ligament

Bone

Bone

Cartilage covers end of bone

Ligament is fibrous tissue that holds bones together

Synovial membrane lines joint capsule and produces synovial fluid

Synovial fluid lubricates joint

Seven cervical vertebrae form neck

12 thoracic vertebrae support ribcage

Five lumbar vertebrae form lower back

Intervertebral discs cushion vertebrae

Sacrum (five fused vertebrae)

Coccyx, or tailbone (four fused vertebrae)

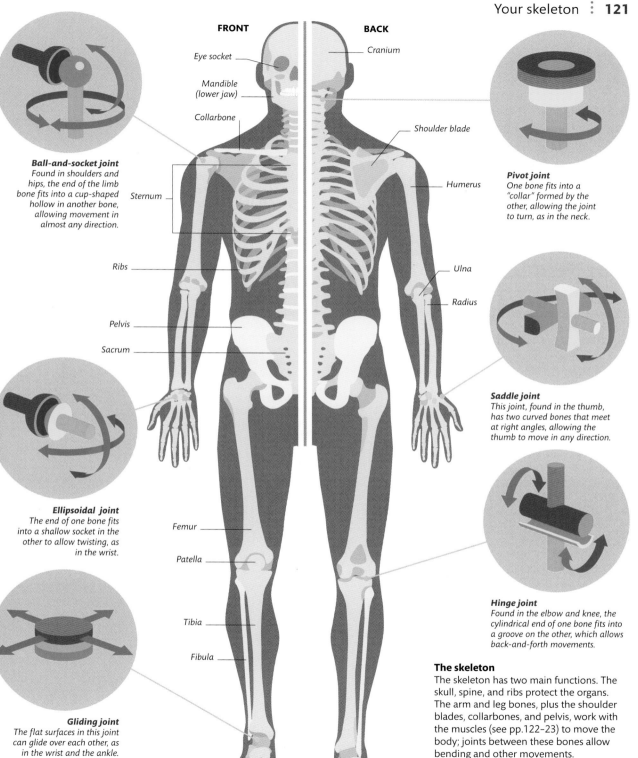

FRONT

BACK

Eye socket

Cranium

Mandible
(lower jaw)

Collarbone

Shoulder blade

Ball-and-socket joint
*Found in shoulders and
hips, the end of the limb
bone fits into a cup-shaped
hollow in another bone,
allowing movement in
almost any direction.*

Sternum

Humerus

Pivot joint
*One bone fits into a
"collar" formed by the
other, allowing the joint
to turn, as in the neck.*

Ribs

Pelvis

Ulna

Radius

Sacrum

Saddle joint
*This joint, found in the thumb,
has two curved bones that meet
at right angles, allowing the
thumb to move in any direction.*

Ellipsoidal joint
*The end of one bone fits
into a shallow socket in the
other to allow twisting, as
in the wrist.*

Femur

Patella

Hinge joint
*Found in the elbow and knee, the
cylindrical end of one bone fits into
a groove on the other, which allows
back-and-forth movements.*

Tibia

Fibula

The skeleton
The skeleton has two main functions. The
skull, spine, and ribs protect the organs.
The arm and leg bones, plus the shoulder
blades, collarbones, and pelvis, work with
the muscles (see pp.122–23) to move the
body; joints between these bones allow
bending and other movements.

Gliding joint
*The flat surfaces in this joint
can glide over each other, as
in the wrist and the ankle.*

Your muscles

The bones of your skeleton (see pp.120–21) are moved by muscles – bundles of tissue that contract to pull on a bone. Keeping your skeleton, muscles, and connective tissues healthy will ensure that you can move freely and minimize your risk of injuries.

The masseter muscle in your jaw is the strongest muscle in the body for its size

CHECKING MUSCULAR AND SKELETAL HEALTH

You are unlikely to need checks if you are healthy, but as you age, you lose bone density and muscle mass, which can lead to a loss of strength and risk of arthritis and fractures. To check your musculoskeletal function, the doctor may ask you how easily you can do daily activities. He or she may ask you to walk a few paces or may check your grip strength. If you have pain or stiffness, you may need an X-ray or a bone scan, or blood tests to detect calcium (resulting from excess bone breakdown) or chemicals resulting from muscle damage.

Muscles and movement

Muscles cannot push, they can only pull, so each joint needs a pair – one muscle to bend (flex) the joint and another to straighten (extend) it. As one muscle contracts, the opposite muscle relaxes. Each muscle stretches across the joint; it is attached to one bone at the end furthest from the joint, and to the other bone just beyond the joint. For example, the muscles of the upper arm are attached at the shoulder and stretch across the elbow to attach to the bones of the forearm.

Muscle attachment

Muscles are attached to bones by strong, fibrous tissues called tendons. The ends of each tendon are anchored in the outer layer of the bone. Most tendons do not stretch, so when the muscle contracts, the bone is forced to move.

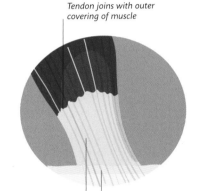

Tendon joins with outer covering of muscle

Tendon formed from sheets or cords of tough collagen fibre

End of tendon embedded in outer layer of bone

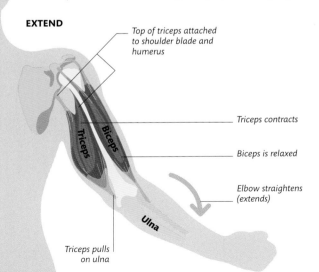

FLEX

Biceps contracts, pulling on radius

Shoulder blade

Biceps

Triceps

Radius

Tendon

Humerus

Triceps is relaxed

Elbow bends (flexes)

EXTEND

Top of triceps attached to shoulder blade and humerus

Triceps

Biceps

Triceps contracts

Biceps is relaxed

Elbow straightens (extends)

Ulna

Triceps pulls on ulna

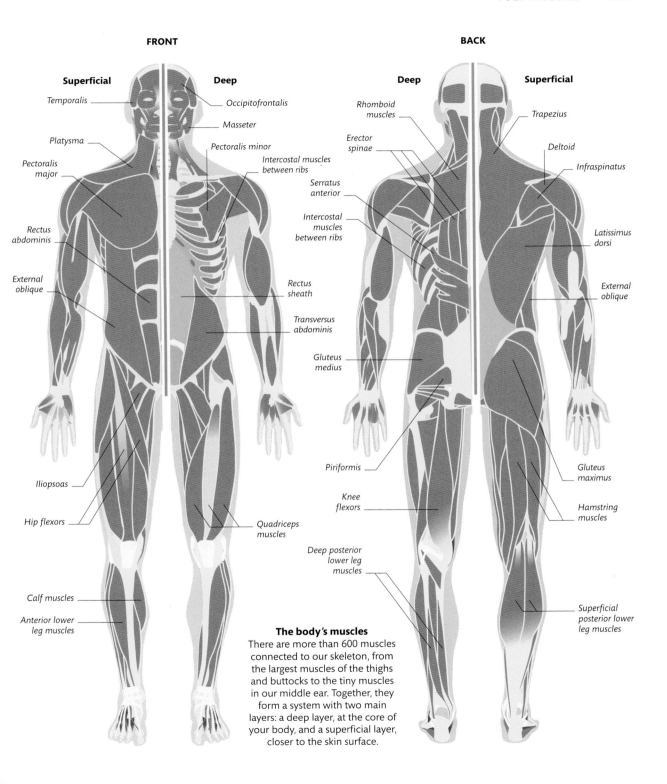

FRONT

Superficial | **Deep**

- Temporalis
- Occipitofrontalis
- Masseter
- Platysma
- Pectoralis minor
- Pectoralis major
- Intercostal muscles between ribs
- Rectus abdominis
- External oblique
- Rectus sheath
- Transversus abdominis
- Iliopsoas
- Hip flexors
- Quadriceps muscles
- Calf muscles
- Anterior lower leg muscles

BACK

Deep | **Superficial**

- Rhomboid muscles
- Trapezius
- Erector spinae
- Deltoid
- Serratus anterior
- Infraspinatus
- Intercostal muscles between ribs
- Latissimus dorsi
- External oblique
- Gluteus medius
- Piriformis
- Gluteus maximus
- Knee flexors
- Hamstring muscles
- Deep posterior lower leg muscles
- Superficial posterior lower leg muscles

The body's muscles

There are more than 600 muscles connected to our skeleton, from the largest muscles of the thighs and buttocks to the tiny muscles in our middle ear. Together, they form a system with two main layers: a deep layer, at the core of your body, and a superficial layer, closer to the skin surface.

Flexibility, posture, and gait

Assessing your flexibility, posture, and gait can provide useful insight into an existing condition, identify if you are at risk of developing chronic joint pain, and monitor improvements gained from training or rehabilitation programmes.

Testing your flexibility

Flexibility is the ability to move a joint through its range of motion. It is determined by your bony anatomy and how well your muscles, tendons, and ligaments work around the joint. There are several ways to assess your general flexibility, as well as the flexibility of specific joints or groups of joints. The sit-and-reach test (below) is commonly used to assess the trunk, pelvis, and hamstrings. Other tests, include the "back–scratch" test to assess shoulder flexibility, and the femoral stretch, or Ely test, to assess the quadriceps in the thigh. A brief warm-up will improve the results and reliability of your flexibility assessment. Results are compared to those predicted for your age and sex and reported as excellent, good, fair, or poor.

ARE YOU TOO FLEXIBLE?

Too much flexibility, due, for instance, to excess elasticity in the tendons, can result in weak and unstable joints, or hypermobility. The Beighton score is a self-test that assesses hypermobility according to the number of "yes" answers to flexibility questions. Your score is your total number of "yes" answers to five questions, each applied to both sides of the body. Pictured below are two of the five questions.

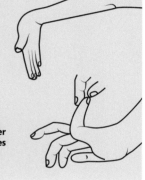

Can you bend your elbow backwards more than 10 degrees?

Can you bend your little finger up at 90 degrees to the back of your hand?

Are you flexible enough?
In the sit-and-reach test, the legs are straight and the feet pressed firmly against the measuring box. The distance reached is recorded and monitored for improvement over time.

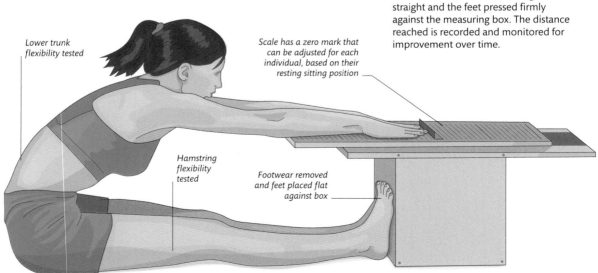

Lower trunk flexibility tested

Scale has a zero mark that can be adjusted for each individual, based on their resting sitting position

Hamstring flexibility tested

Footwear removed and feet placed flat against box

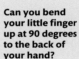

Assessing your posture

Posture refers to your body alignment as you stand or sit. For good posture, your muscles need to hold your skeleton so it is balanced, with your spine straight but fairly relaxed. Abnormal posture may result from illness, injury, or habitual behaviour, and can cause muscle imbalance and chronic joint pain. To assess your posture, you will be asked to stand (or, less commonly, sit) while the assessor examines you from the front, side, and back. Mild postural errors, such as slouching, are common and often easily correctable. Severe postural abnormalities may require further investigation or treatment by a doctor or physiotherapist.

Assessing your gait

Your gait, or your pattern of walking, is influenced by muscular strength, balance, and flexibility. It evolves from childhood to old age and is affected by illness and injuries. Gait consists of the stance phase and swing phase, each of which can be analysed. Conventional gait assessment involves taking steps on a flat surface or treadmill. The assessor observes aspects of each phase and also inspects your shoes for wear distribution. Gait laboratories can conduct deeper analysis using optical tracking systems, force plates, and electromyography (EMG). Wearable technology may also be used to measure gait parameters.

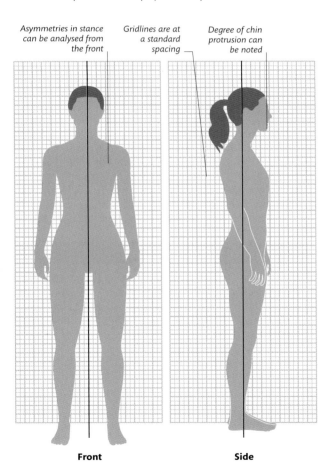

Asymmetries in stance can be analysed from the front

Gridlines are at a standard spacing

Degree of chin protrusion can be noted

Front

Side

Postural analysis
A postural analysis grid chart may help the assessor to identify abnormalities, such as kyphosis, scoliosis, or hyperlordosis, which are abnormal spinal curvatures. A plumbline can be used in combination with the grid.

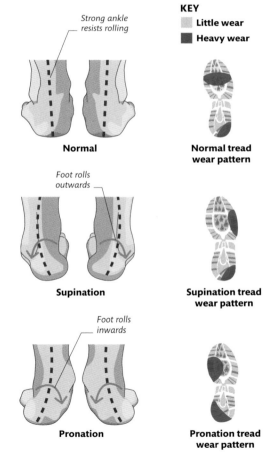

KEY

☐ **Little wear**

■ **Heavy wear**

Strong ankle resists rolling

Normal

Normal tread wear pattern

Foot rolls outwards

Supination

Supination tread wear pattern

Foot rolls inwards

Pronation

Pronation tread wear pattern

Ankle rotation
Patterns such as pronation (foot rolls inwards in stance phase) and supination (foot rolls outwards in stance phase) may be identified by gait analysis. These conditions require appropriate supportive footwear.

Core components

The core comprises many elements of the musculoskeletal system. These include superficial muscles, such as gluteal and abdominal muscles (see p.123), and deep muscles, such as the pelvic floor and diaphragm, that stabilize and strengthen body structures.

Multifidus – a key deep stabilizing muscle of the spine

Diaphragm – a strong muscular roof to the abdomen

Transversus abdominis – the innermost of three sheet-like abdominal muscles

Sacrum – anchors some deep core stabilizing muscles

Pelvic floor – a sheet of muscle that supports the organs above

Multifidus

Diaphragm

Transversus abdominis

Sacrum

Pelvic floor

Core stability testing

Your musculoskeletal core provides a stable foundation for all your limb movements, including activities of daily living, recreation, or sport. Maintaining strength and dynamic control of the core muscles is important for preventing injuries and for building strength in exercise and rehabilitation.

Core stability

The body's core consists of the spine, abdomen, hips, and pelvis, and the core muscles include the paraspinal, abdominal, gluteal, pelvic floor, and hip girdle muscles. Improving core stability requires training that focuses not only on strength, but also endurance, flexibility, and dynamic coordination of the active (muscles) and passive (bones and ligaments) components of the core. While a stable core provides a foundation for all movements, core instability can be implicated in numerous chronic musculoskeletal conditions.

MAINTAINING CORE STABILITY

Core stability exercises can be performed without special equipment. You can build them into your daily routine to develop a strong foundation for your body. Begin with short intervals of forearm planks (body straight, facing down with elbows on the ground) and side planks (see opposite). Gradually increase duration as stability improves. Try the "bird-dog": start on all fours and raise one limb at a time, progressing to two limbs and increasing duration.

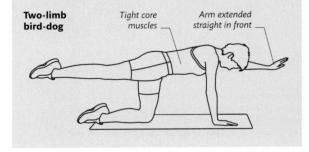

Two-limb bird-dog

Tight core muscles

Arm extended straight in front

Testing core stability

Various tests may be used to assess your core stability, including single-leg squats (see below), the lateral bridge, and the torso flexor and extensor endurance tests (see right). In these last three tests, you have to hold a specific posture for as long as you can; this period can then be compared to values from healthy individuals, or to repeat measurements taken during training or rehabilitation programmes to monitor progress.

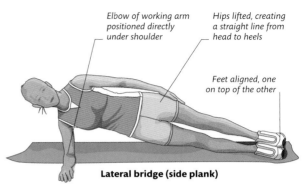

Elbow of working arm positioned directly under shoulder

Hips lifted, creating a straight line from head to heels

Feet aligned, one on top of the other

Lateral bridge (side plank)

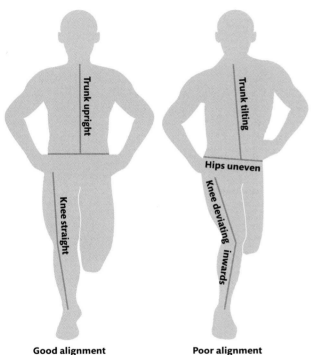

Trunk upright

Knee straight

Good alignment

Trunk tilting

Hips uneven

Knee deviating inwards

Poor alignment

Single-leg squat

In this exercise, you stand on one leg, with your body straight, and then lower your body. It tests control and coordination of your hip and trunk muscles. If you struggle to keep your body straight and your pelvis level, this may indicate core instability.

⏱ **Average, fit 21-year-olds can hold the lateral bridge for 95 seconds (men) or 75 seconds (women)**

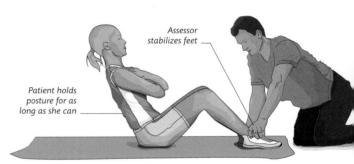

Assessor stabilizes feet

Patient holds posture for as long as she can

Torso flexor endurance

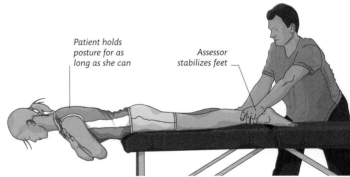

Patient holds posture for as long as she can

Assessor stabilizes feet

Torso extensor endurance

Common tests

The lateral bridge (also known as side plank) and the torso flexor and extensor endurance tests are timed tests to assess the strength, endurance, and functional control of the front, back, and side of your core muscles. Often added to these is the prone bridge (or straight plank), which is similar to a push-up except that the forearms and hands are kept flat against the floor.

Muscle strength and endurance

Strength and endurance are key components of muscle fitness. Building your muscles provides benefits such as improved bone mass, blood glucose control, and the ability to perform everyday activities easily. Testing muscle fitness provides information on your baseline function and identifies aspects that may benefit from targeted training.

Muscle strength

The strength of a particular muscle or muscle group is typically measured by tests in which you have to push or pull against resistance. Strength tests may be static (in which you contract your muscles without moving your limb) or dynamic (in which you move your limb to counter the resistance). The tests may involve pushing against a hard surface; resisting pressure from a doctor's or therapist's hands; or pushing or pulling against a machine. To achieve reliable results, it is helpful to warm up before the test, and begin with a weight or resistance that is 50–70 per cent of your expected capacity, increasing gradually. For safety and reliability, you should use a spotter, whose role includes assisting with a lift that is beyond your ability. Results are adjusted for body weight for comparability.

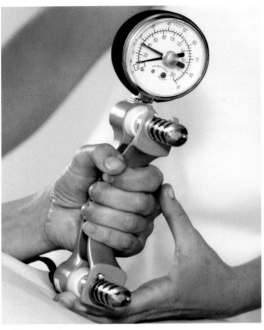

Grip strength
A dynamometer can be used to measure grip strength. This is an example of a static resistance test. A 5-kg (11-lb) reduction in grip strength may be associated with an increased risk of illnesses such as cardiovascular disease.

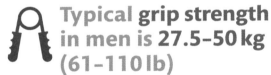

Typical grip strength in men is 27.5–50 kg (61–110 lb)

Legpress

Dynamic strength tests include the benchpress for upper body and legpress for lower body muscle strength. The pictured machine is designed for the 45-degree legpress.

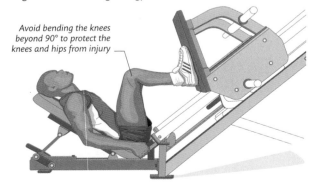

Avoid bending the knees beyond 90° to protect the knees and hips from injury

❶ Legs flexed

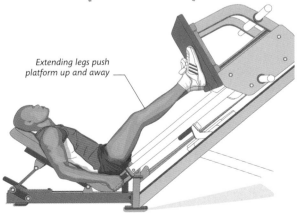

Extending legs push platform up and away

❷ Legs extended

Muscle endurance

Muscle endurance is the ability of a muscle or group of muscles to maintain a contraction or perform repeated contractions against resistance over a period of time. This provides information on muscle function and control.

The maximum number of push-ups or curl-ups performed without rest are simple tests that may be used to evaluate upper body and abdominal muscle endurance. Resistance exercises, such as the benchpress and legpress, can be adapted for endurance testing by finding your maximum number of repetitions with a specific weight. Testing muscle endurance provides insight into muscle fitness and fatigue, identifies areas in need of specific training, and may be used to diagnose or monitor some neuromuscular conditions.

Curl-up endurance

In average people, the number of curl-ups achieved varies from 27–31 in your twenties to 13–19 in your sixties. Arm position should be standardized for comparability – arms could also be crossed over the chest or pointing towards the feet.

RESISTANCE TRAINING

For effective resistance training, you need suitable exercises for your fitness level, gradual progression, adequate rest and nutrition, supervision, and appropriate professional advice. "Open-chain" exercises, such as leg extension, are performed in non-weight-bearing positions, where your limb can move freely against resistance. In "closed-chain" exercises, such as lunges, your hands and feet are fixed in weight-bearing positions and the movement involves coordination of multiple joints. Resistance training usually involves both types of exercise, but closed-chain exercises put less stress on your joints.

**Lunge
(closed-chain exercise)**

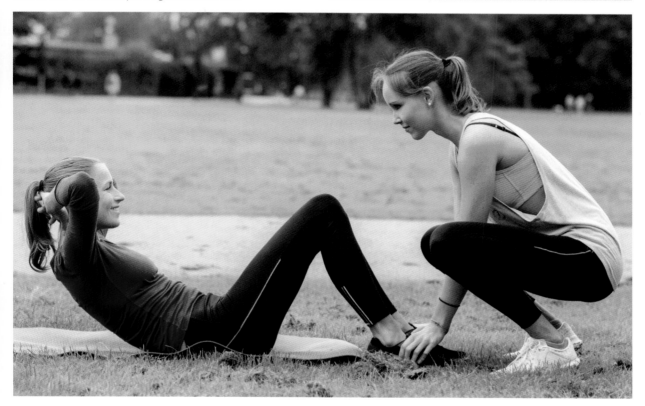

Your nervous system

The nervous system forms the communication system in your body. It comprises a network of nerve cells that transmits hundreds of electrical signals per second to control all of your physical and mental functions, from your breathing and heartbeat to complex thought.

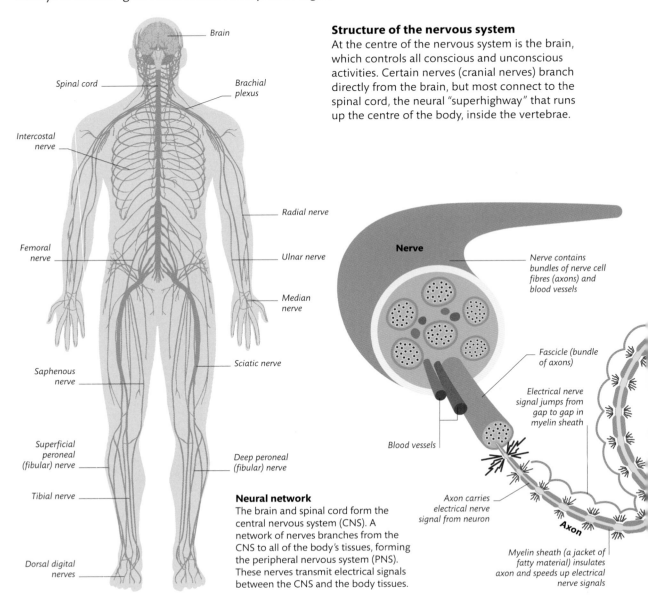

Brain

Spinal cord

Brachial plexus

Intercostal nerve

Radial nerve

Femoral nerve

Ulnar nerve

Median nerve

Saphenous nerve

Sciatic nerve

Superficial peroneal (fibular) nerve

Deep peroneal (fibular) nerve

Tibial nerve

Dorsal digital nerves

Nerve

Nerve contains bundles of nerve cell fibres (axons) and blood vessels

Fascicle (bundle of axons)

Electrical nerve signal jumps from gap to gap in myelin sheath

Blood vessels

Axon carries electrical nerve signal from neuron

Axon

Myelin sheath (a jacket of fatty material) insulates axon and speeds up electrical nerve signals

Structure of the nervous system

At the centre of the nervous system is the brain, which controls all conscious and unconscious activities. Certain nerves (cranial nerves) branch directly from the brain, but most connect to the spinal cord, the neural "superhighway" that runs up the centre of the body, inside the vertebrae.

Neural network

The brain and spinal cord form the central nervous system (CNS). A network of nerves branches from the CNS to all of the body's tissues, forming the peripheral nervous system (PNS). These nerves transmit electrical signals between the CNS and the body tissues.

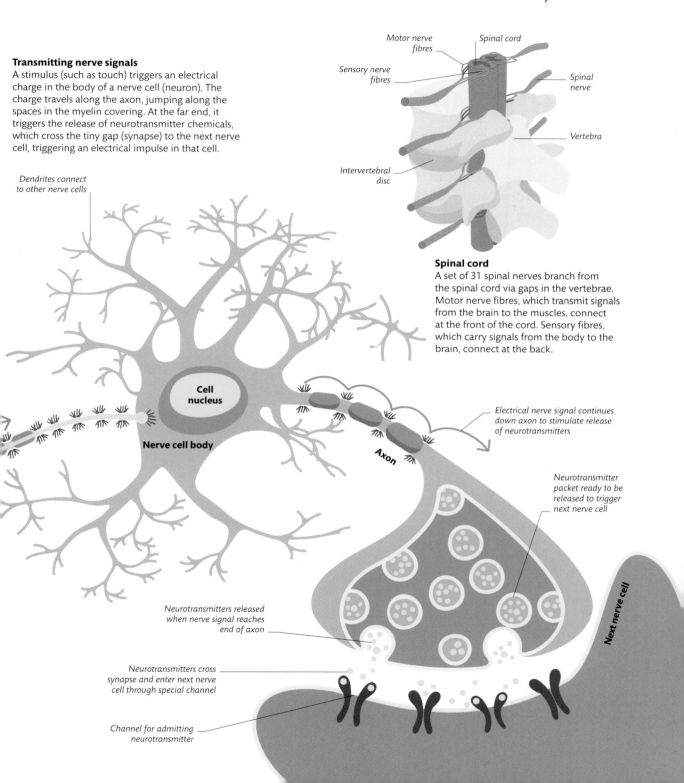

Transmitting nerve signals

A stimulus (such as touch) triggers an electrical charge in the body of a nerve cell (neuron). The charge travels along the axon, jumping along the spaces in the myelin covering. At the far end, it triggers the release of neurotransmitter chemicals, which cross the tiny gap (synapse) to the next nerve cell, triggering an electrical impulse in that cell.

Motor nerve fibres

Sensory nerve fibres

Spinal cord

Spinal nerve

Vertebra

Intervertebral disc

Dendrites connect to other nerve cells

Spinal cord

A set of 31 spinal nerves branch from the spinal cord via gaps in the vertebrae. Motor nerve fibres, which transmit signals from the brain to the muscles, connect at the front of the cord. Sensory fibres, which carry signals from the body to the brain, connect at the back.

Cell nucleus

Nerve cell body

Axon

Electrical nerve signal continues down axon to stimulate release of neurotransmitters

Neurotransmitter packet ready to be released to trigger next nerve cell

Next nerve cell

Neurotransmitters released when nerve signal reaches end of axon

Neurotransmitters cross synapse and enter next nerve cell through special channel

Channel for admitting neurotransmitter

How your nervous system works

The nervous system functions in two main ways. It enables you to make deliberate, conscious movements. It also carries out the unconscious activities that keep you alive, such as regulating your breathing and heartbeat and producing rapid reflex actions.

Inputs and outputs

Both voluntary and involuntary actions result from messages passing along the nerves between the body tissues and central nervous system (brain and spinal cord). Sensory nerves send information about changes outside or inside the body to the central nervous system, which processes the information and sends out response signals along motor nerves.

Nerve signals can travel at speeds of up to 120 m per second (390 ft per second)

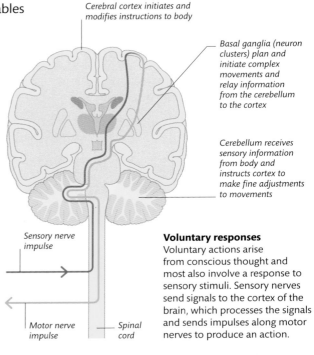

Cerebral cortex initiates and modifies instructions to body

Basal ganglia (neuron clusters) plan and initiate complex movements and relay information from the cerebellum to the cortex

Cerebellum receives sensory information from body and instructs cortex to make fine adjustments to movements

Sensory nerve impulse

Motor nerve impulse

Spinal cord

Voluntary responses

Voluntary actions arise from conscious thought and most also involve a response to sensory stimuli. Sensory nerves send signals to the cortex of the brain, which processes the signals and sends impulses along motor nerves to produce an action.

The autonomic nervous system

The autonomic nervous system involves the whole body. It has two parts: the sympathetic system and the parasympathetic system. Each of the two systems produces a different response in a particular part of the body. In general, the sympathetic system prepares the body for action or to cope with stress – the "fight or flight" reaction. The parasympathetic system acts to help conserve or restore energy.

Part of body affected	Sympathetic response	Parasympathetic response
Eyes	• Pupils widen • Tear production decreases	• Pupils constrict • Tear production increases
Mouth	• Saliva production decreases	• Saliva production increases
Digestive system	• Movement of food through intestine slows down • Production of digestive enzymes decreases	• Movement of food through intestine speeds up • Production of digestive enzymes increases

CHECKING THE NERVOUS SYSTEM

Some changes that affect the nervous system, such as slower reactions, are just a part of normal ageing. However, some symptoms, such as tingling in your hands and feet or difficulties with your balance, could be early indications of an underlying condition and should be checked by a doctor.

To test your nervous system, the doctor may first carry out simple tests, such as checking your reflexes, coordination, and senses. If the results of these tests indicate a health problem, you may be advised to have other investigations, such as tests of the electrical activity in your brain or muscles.

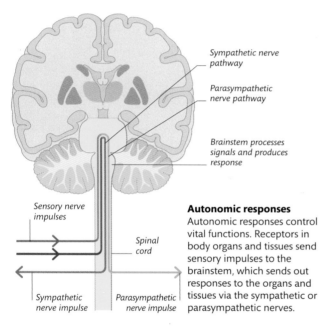

Sympathetic nerve pathway

Parasympathetic nerve pathway

Brainstem processes signals and produces response

Sensory nerve impulses

Spinal cord

Sympathetic nerve impulse

Parasympathetic nerve impulse

Autonomic responses
Autonomic responses control vital functions. Receptors in body organs and tissues send sensory impulses to the brainstem, which sends out responses to the organs and tissues via the sympathetic or parasympathetic nerves.

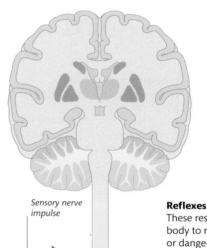

Sensory nerve impulse

Motor nerve impulse

Spinal cord

Reflexes
These responses enable the body to react instantly to pain or danger. Signals from sensory nerves do not reach the brain; instead, they are processed by the spinal cord, which sends responses directly to the appropriate body muscles.

Part of body affected	Sympathetic response	Parasympathetic response	Part of body affected	Sympathetic response	Parasympathetic response
Blood vessels	• Arteries to muscles and brain widen; arteries to skin and digestive tract narrow	• Arteries to muscles, brain, skin, and digestive tract return to normal size	Adrenal glands	• Release adrenaline and noradrenaline	• Reduce production of adrenaline and noradrenaline
Heart	• Heartbeat speeds up	• Heartbeat slows down	Skin	• Sweat production increases	• Sweat production decreases
Lungs	• Airways widen	• Airways narrow	Urinary system	• Kidneys reduce urine output • Bladder neck squeezes shut	• Kidneys increase urine output • Bladder neck relaxes

Testing your reflexes

Reflexes are simple involuntary, or automatic, muscle reactions to stimuli that are activated to protect you from environmental dangers: for example, by quickly withdrawing your hand when it nears a flame.

What to expect when tested

When sensory nerves detect danger they send a message to the spinal cord, and corresponding motor nerves carry a response straight to the relevant muscles, bypassing the brain. Doctors test certain reflexes to check that pathways are complete. They generally begin by looking at reflexes in the lower limbs as they are furthest from the spinal cord, and then look at the upper body if impairment is detected.

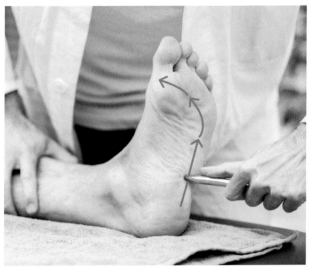

Babinski foot reflex test
A doctor will gently but firmly stroke the outer edge of the sole of your foot, from the heel to the base of the big toe. In a normal reaction all your toes will point down together.

Testing coordination and balance

Critical to injury prevention, balance (the ability to maintain a position) and coordination (the capacity to execute sets of movements smoothly) depend on complex interactions between organs such as the eyes and ears and many different body systems.

How both are assessed

Your doctor will start with a physical examination that includes checking your eyes and ears, then ask you to perform some tests. To assess balance you may be asked to walk in a straight line, touching the heel of one foot to the toe of the other with each step, and/or stand on one leg (see right) – with your eyes open, then closed.

Coordination tests might include the finger-to-nose test (see opposite). You may be asked to draw a circle with each big toe or index finger. To assess leg coordination you may sit or lie down and put the heel of one foot on your other knee and attempt to slide the heel down your shin towards the ankle. If the tests reveal abnormalities you will be referred for further tests.

BALANCING TEST

Stand on one leg (near a wall or chair in case you need support). Try to hold the position for a minute, first with your eyes open and then with them shut. Repeat with the other leg.

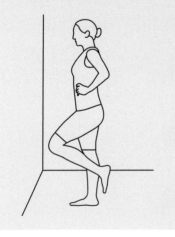

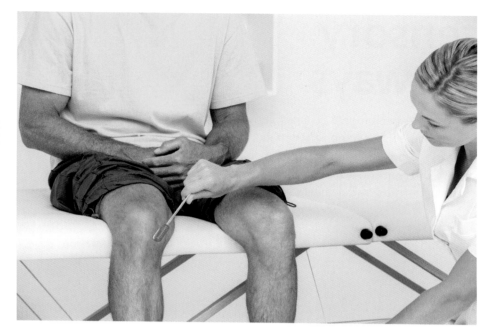

Assessing the knee reflex
While you sit on a chair or the edge of a bed with your legs hanging down, your doctor will give a sharp tap to the tendon just below the knee cap. In response, the muscles over the front of the upper leg should contract, causing the leg to "kick".

Nose-to-finger test
Your doctor will hold out a finger and ask you to focus on their face and then touch their finger, then your nose, then the finger again. You will be asked to repeat this several times as fast you can.

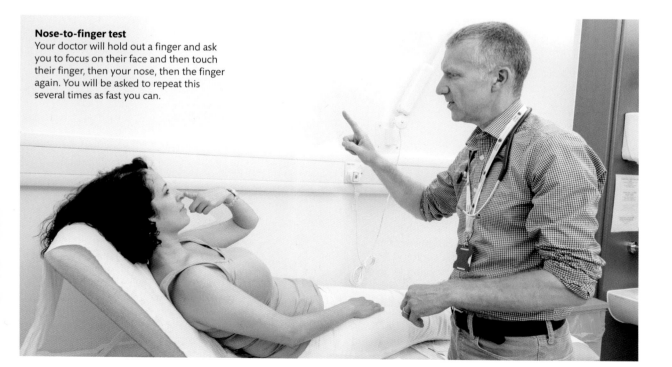

Testing sensory nerve pathways

Injury and some medical conditions, most commonly diabetes, can result in peripheral neuropathy – damage to the peripheral nerves. This damage typically causes weakness and numbness in the area of the body supplied by those nerves. The type and extent of the damage varies depending on the functions performed by the affected nerves.

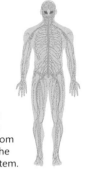

Peripheral nerves
The sensory nerves carry vital signals from the extremities to the central nervous system.

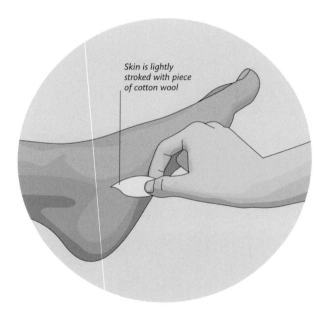

Skin is lightly stroked with piece of cotton wool

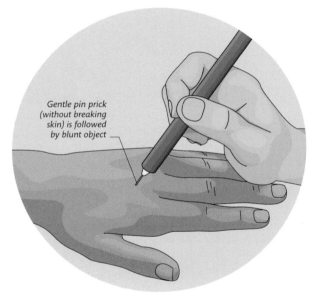

Gentle pin prick (without breaking skin) is followed by blunt object

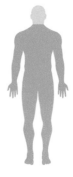

Light-touch test
This tests for areas of insensitivity that might indicate a lesion affecting a peripheral nerve. The doctor will show you what they are going to do at a point where you can feel it, then test other parts of your body, so that they can map areas of insensitivity. Your doctor will gently stroke your skin with cotton wool and ask you to describe what you can feel.

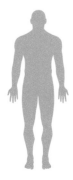

Pain-type test
Also known as the pin-prick test, this involves touching your skin alternately with a sharp, pin-like object, then a blunt one, such as a round pinhead. You will be asked to identify whether it is sharp or blunt – the aim is to find out if you can tell the difference. Your doctor will compare both sides of the body and, depending on the reasons for testing, may work from the feet up, or start further up the body.

WHAT HAPPENS DURING THE TESTS

Your doctor may undertake a number of checks to gain a complete picture because, although the sensations share the same spinal cord pathway, each one arises from different nerve receptors and terminates in a different part of the brain. They will probably ask you to lie down for these assessments and you will need to close your eyes for each test so that you cannot anticipate the stimuli. Your doctor will compare both sides of the body, and is most likely to start with the feet and legs because these nerve pathways are longest and the first to show any loss of sensation. If sensory loss is detected, you may be referred to a specialist for further tests.

Persistent high blood sugar levels can lead to nerve damage

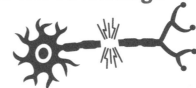

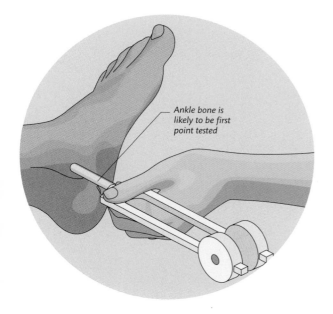

Ankle bone is likely to be first point tested

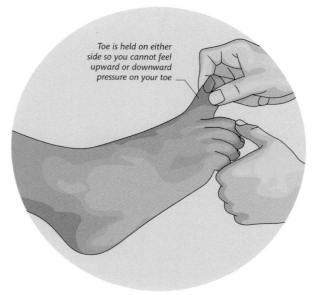

Toe is held on either side so you cannot feel upward or downward pressure on your toe

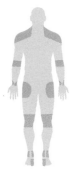

Vibration sensation

Vibratory sensation travels to the brain via the same pathways as those for position sense (see right) and may be diminished in people with peripheral neuropathy. Your doctor will strike a tuning fork against a hard surface, then hold it against a point where the bone is close to the surface and ask you to say whether or not you feel the vibration, and if you can, when it stops.

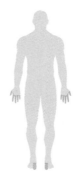

Position sense

This technique assesses your body's ability to know where it is in space, also known as proprioception: a factor critical to balance. Supporting your foot, your doctor will hold either side of your big toe, then move it up and down, asking you to describe where your toe is. The test will be done on both feet; depending on the findings, it may be repeated on your fingers.

How your mind works

Your mind is responsible for conscious thoughts and actions, learning, and memory. These tasks involve taking in signals from the outside world, via nerves in the rest of the body, and integrating them with information already stored in the brain.

Centres of brain activity
Some parts of the cortex process nerve signals from other parts of the body, such as the eyes, ears, and skin. Other areas generate conscious actions, such as speech and coordinated movements. Certain regions, called association areas, integrate new information with existing memories and emotions.

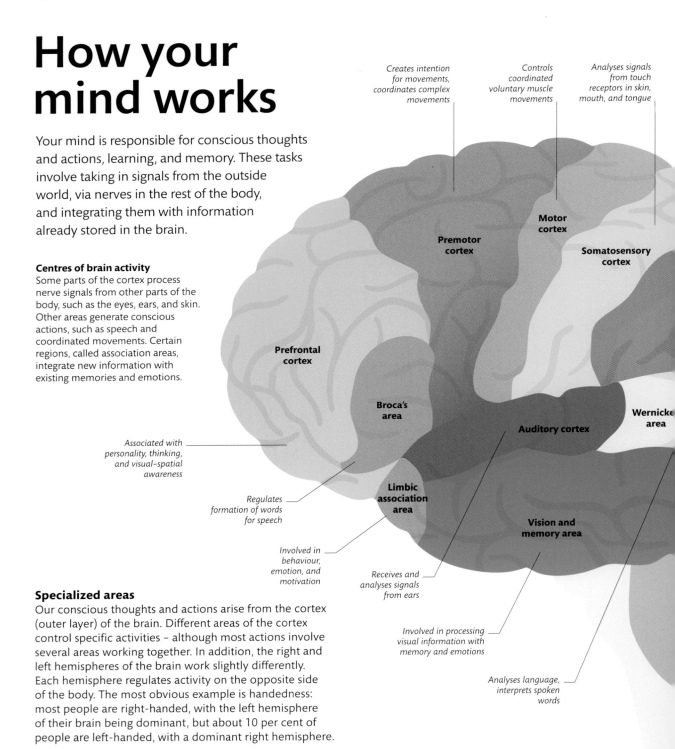

Creates intention for movements, coordinates complex movements

Controls coordinated voluntary muscle movements

Analyses signals from touch receptors in skin, mouth, and tongue

Motor cortex

Premotor cortex

Somatosensory cortex

Prefrontal cortex

Broca's area

Wernicke area

Auditory cortex

Associated with personality, thinking, and visual–spatial awareness

Regulates formation of words for speech

Limbic association area

Vision and memory area

Involved in behaviour, emotion, and motivation

Receives and analyses signals from ears

Involved in processing visual information with memory and emotions

Analyses language, interprets spoken words

Specialized areas
Our conscious thoughts and actions arise from the cortex (outer layer) of the brain. Different areas of the cortex control specific activities – although most actions involve several areas working together. In addition, the right and left hemispheres of the brain work slightly differently. Each hemisphere regulates activity on the opposite side of the body. The most obvious example is handedness: most people are right-handed, with the left hemisphere of their brain being dominant, but about 10 per cent of people are left-handed, with a dominant right hemisphere.

Memory storage

The creation, storage, and recall of memories involve several areas of the brain. The cortex processes information, while the hippocampus converts perceptions and thoughts into longer-term memories. The amygdala registers emotions, which give significance to our memories.

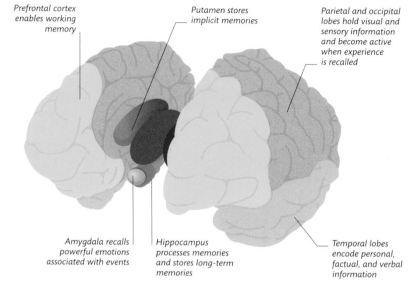

Prefrontal cortex enables working memory

Putamen stores implicit memories

Parietal and occipital lobes hold visual and sensory information and become active when experience is recalled

Amygdala recalls powerful emotions associated with events

Hippocampus processes memories and stores long-term memories

Temporal lobes encode personal, factual, and verbal information

Integrates general sensory information

Sensory association cortex

Visual association cortex

Integrates visual information with other sensory information, memory, and emotions

Primary visual cortex

Receives and analyses signals from the eyes

Cerebellum

Coordinates bodily movements through control of muscles

The **record** for learning to speak a **new language** is just **1 hour 40 minutes**

Learning and memory

Memory is not just about storing data; memories are also recalled and integrated with new information. There are different forms of memory, for specific tasks. Working memory holds information only as long as you need it. Declarative memories comprise factual knowledge and ideas. Episodic memories involve personal experiences. Spatial memories provide a map of your environment. Implicit memories are learned information that you can use without conscious effort, such as knowing how to drive.

CHECKING MENTAL FUNCTION

To assess your mental health, the doctor will ask you about your lifestyle – diet, sleep, alcohol or drug use, and possible sources of stress. If necessary, the doctor may also assess your risk of more serious conditions such as depression or dementia, typically by using a standardized questionnaire.

Mood analysis

Many people experience times when they feel low, but it is vital to see your doctor if you suffer from severe anxiety, or you have been feeling sad and "down" for weeks or months (depression), as both can impact on daily life.

What to expect when consulting your doctor

Your doctor will ask you some standard questions about your mood, behaviour, thoughts, and lifestyle, and will want to know about any changes in the quality of these aspects of your life as well as events that might have triggered your feelings. You will be asked to describe how you feel, and how long you have felt this way, as well as physical factors that affect you, such as disturbed sleep, unexplained aches and pains, panic attacks, or comfort eating. Your doctor will also want to know if your mood impinges on social aspects of your life such as your work or relationships with others and, if so, to what extent.

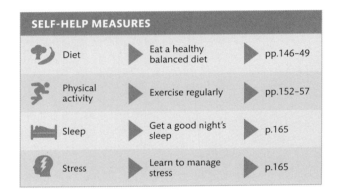

SELF-HELP MEASURES		
Diet	Eat a healthy balanced diet	pp.146–49
Physical activity	Exercise regularly	pp.152–57
Sleep	Get a good night's sleep	p.165
Stress	Learn to manage stress	p.165

Dementia testing

Dementia is not a specific disease, but a term used to describe a group of symptoms associated with a decline in mental ability – memory and thinking skills – as well as behaviour severe enough to interfere with your ability to perform everyday tasks.

What happens in the consultation?

Your doctor will want to know when you first became aware of the symptoms, how they are affecting you, and whether there is any family history of memory impairment. You may be asked to complete a cognitive test that assesses mental abilities, such as memory, concentration, and language skills, as well as behaviour and visual perception.

This will include questions such as what is today's date or day of the week, and where did you go to school. There will be some basic maths calculations, as well as drawing tests, image identification, and problem-solving tasks. There are online sites that provide similar questionnaires you can use to assess cognitive functioning at home – but always show the doctor your results. Your doctor will also conduct a physical examination, review any medications, and may request blood tests to exclude conditions with symptoms that can be confused with dementia.

From these tests your doctor can assess whether or not your impairment is a normal part of the ageing process or associated with dementia. You may also be referred for brain scans to assess the cause of the symptoms.

More than 46 million people are living with dementia worldwide

The next steps

Low mood, anxiety, or depression can reduce your desire for exercise and increase the likelihood of comfort eating, or even alcohol and drug abuse, leaving you more at risk of physical problems. Your doctor will conduct an examination and may order blood tests (see p.54) to eliminate any illnesses that could be the cause of mood changes. Depending on the findings, self-help measures (left) and referral for talking therapies may be suggested.

1 in 10 people suffer from depression at some point in their lives

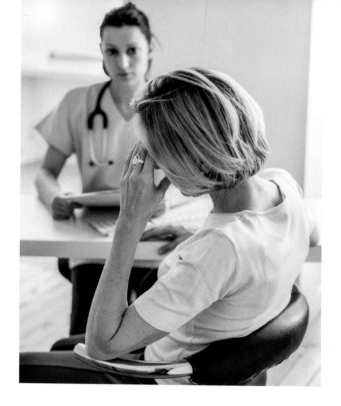

Talking to your doctor

Opening up and telling your doctor about how you really feel can be difficult, but it is essential to be honest so that he or she get a full picture and can be in a position to offer the right help.

DIFFERENTIATING BETWEEN AGE-RELATED CHANGES AND DEMENTIA

Age-related changes	Signs and symptoms of dementia
Occasionally forgetting words, names, or events, but recalling them later. Cannot remember a conversation that took place a year ago	Forgetting recently learned information, conversations, or a recent event. Repeatedly telling the same story or asking the same question
Occasionally becoming confused about the day of the week	Losing track of days, dates, and seasons. Forgetting where you are or even how you got there
Intermittent loss of interest in regular activities, family, or work, which are normally enjoyed	Starting to withdraw completely from favourite pastimes, social groups, and regular activities
Occasionally making poor decisions or showing lack of judgement	Persistent poor financial judgement, loss of interest in personal care
Sometimes losing possessions, but able to retrace steps to find them	Putting items in unusual places and and inability to retrace steps to find them; you may accuse others of stealing your possessions
Developing age-related vision problems such as cataracts	Cannot differentiate colours or detect movement and "sees" things that are not there
Occasionally needing help with familiar tasks such as resetting a clock or recording TV programmes	Is no longer able to complete normally familiar tasks
Sometimes making errors calculating finances	Unable to work with numbers and follow plans/instructions/recipes
Developing routines and specific ways of doing things and becoming irritable if routine is disrupted	Becoming generally confused, suspicious of others, depressed, fearful, and easily upset for no reason

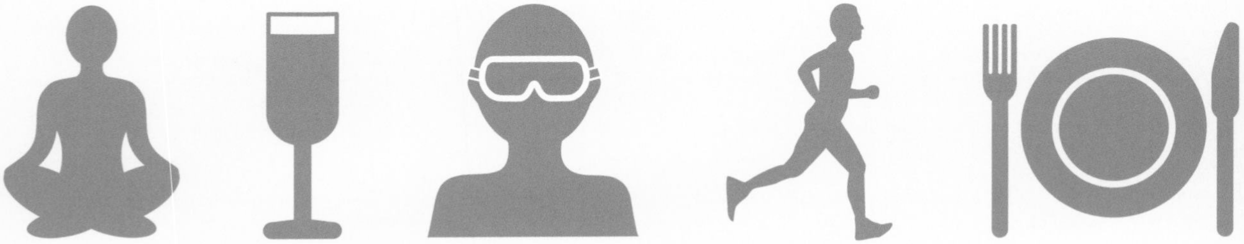

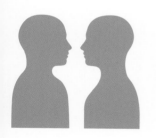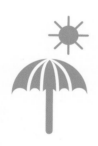 # Optimizing
your health

Vaccinations

Vaccination is an effective method of protecting against a range of potentially serious infectious diseases. Many vaccines are offered as part of the routine vaccination schedule but some are offered only to special groups or at particular ages. In addition, boosters or additional vaccines may be recommended for travel.

How does vaccination work?

A vaccine is a weakened or killed form of an infectious organism, or a toxin or protein from that organism, that provokes your immune system into producing antibodies (also known as immunoglobulins) against the disease the organism causes.

Some vaccines provide reliable long-term immunity whereas others may not give full protection or the protection may not be long-lasting. For example, influenza vaccines usually protect only against the strains of the virus causing the latest outbreaks of flu. Serious adverse effects of vaccines are rare. However, certain vaccines are not generally recommended for certain groups, such as those with weakened immune systems; your doctor will be able to advise you if any vaccines are not suitable for you.

Vaccines provide active immunity, but it is also possible to create passive immunity by injecting immunoglobulins (antibodies) from humans or animals who have been exposed to the disease. However, immunoglobulins do not stimulate the body to produce its own antibodies, and so their protection is short-lived.

COMMON TRAVEL VACCINATIONS FOR ADULTS

The vaccinations recommended for travel depend on the part of the world you intend to visit. Wherever you plan to go, you should make sure you have been immunized against diphtheria, tetanus, and polio, and have had booster doses if necessary. The table below details the more common travel vaccinations in the UK. However, recommendations may change so you should obtain up-to-date information in plenty of time before you travel, because there may be a time lag before a vaccine becomes fully effective, and because some vaccines require more than one dose to provide full protection.

Infection	How given	Protection from full course
• Cholera	Oral dose	About 60–70 per cent protection against severe disease for up to 2 years
• Hepatitis A	Injection	About 99 per cent protection for 20–30 years
• Hepatitis B	Injection	Over 90 per cent protection; immunity is probably life-long
• Japanese encephalitis	Injection	Over 90 per cent protection; duration of protection is unknown
• Meningitis A, C, W135, and Y	Injection	Protects for up to 5 years
• Rabies	Injection	Degree of protection uncertain and may vary depending on extent and duration of exposure to rabies
• Typhoid	Injection or oral dose	Injection gives over 80 per cent protection for 3 years. Oral dose gives about 75 per cent protection for 3 years
• Yellow fever	Injection	About 90 per cent protection for 10 years

COMMON VACCINATIONS IN THE UK

The table below lists the most common vaccines offered routinely in the UK. Most of the vaccines are given by injection and are offered in childhood. (In this table, a baby is under one year old; a child is aged one to nine; an adolescent is aged 10 to 19; and adults are over 19.) Some vaccines are not offered to everybody, but only to those who are in specific at-risk groups, such as people with certain long-term health conditions or healthcare workers.

Infection	How given	To whom offered
• Diphtheria/tetanus/pertussis (whooping cough)/polio/ Haemophilus influenzae type b/hepatitis B	Injection	Babies
• Pneumococcal infection	Injection	Babies, children, and older adults
• Rotavirus infection	Oral dose	Babies
• Meningitis B	Injection	Babies and children
• Haemophilus influenzae type b/meningitis C	Injection	Children
• Measles/mumps/rubella	Injection	Children
• Influenza	Nasal spray	Children
	Injection	Babies, children (certain groups), and adults (certain groups); pregnant women; and older adults
• Diphtheria/tetanus/pertussis (whooping cough)/polio	Injection	Children
• Human papillomavirus	Injection	Adolescents
• Diphtheria/tetanus/polio	Injection	Adolescents
• Meningitis A, C, W, Y	Injection	Adolescents
• Pertussis (whooping cough)	Injection	Pregnant women
• Shingles	Injection	Older adults
• Tuberculosis	Injection	Babies in areas with a high incidence of TB or with a parent or grandparent born in a country with a high incidence of TB
• Chickenpox	Injection	Non-immune people in close contact with those at risk of serious illness from chickenpox

A healthy diet

The human body requires a range of nutrients in order to function. The food we eat must provide sufficient protein, carbohydrate, fat, fibre, vitamins, minerals, phytonutrients, and water to sustain all physiological functions from energy production, growth, repair, and defence, to cell communication, digestion, cognition, and psychological wellbeing.

The essential nutrients

Protein provides the body with amino acids needed for growth, repair, and energy. Carbohydrates – our main source of energy – also contain fibre, essential for cardiovascular and digestive health. Monounsaturated, polyunsaturated, and saturated fats are important sources of fatty acids.

Essential fatty acids (omega-3 and omega-6) are used in maintaining cell structure, synthesizing hormones, and absorbing vitamins A, D, E, and K. Vitamins and minerals provide antioxidants, and enable the body to perform a wide variety of functions, from hormone production to absorbing and transporting nutrients.

Broccoli contains almost **twice** as much **vitamin C** as an **orange** of the same weight

CARING FOR TEETH AND GUMS

- Brush your teeth at least twice a day to minimize plaque build-up. Clean between your teeth with floss or interdental brushes to keep gums clean. Attend regular dental check-ups (see pp.118–19).

- Use a fluoride toothpaste to help build strong teeth and reduce risk of tooth decay.

- Limit your consumption of sugary food and drinks (including alcohol, see p.150), as sugar is the main cause of tooth decay.

- Foods containing calcium (dairy products, almonds, green leafy vegetables, tinned fish) and phosphorus (eggs, fish, poultry, cheese, wholegrains) promote strong teeth and bones.

- Consume a wide variety of fresh vegetables and fruit containing vitamin C as this is essential for gum health.

Stay hydrated

It is recommended that you drink six to eight glasses of fluid a day, with water as the main source. Milk, tea, coffee, and sugar-free drinks (not fizzy drinks or cordials, as they have a high sugar and calorie content) count too. Limit fruit juices and smoothies to 150ml (5 fl oz) per day (one portion). Limit your intake of alcoholic drinks, because these act as a diuretic and so increase dehydration.

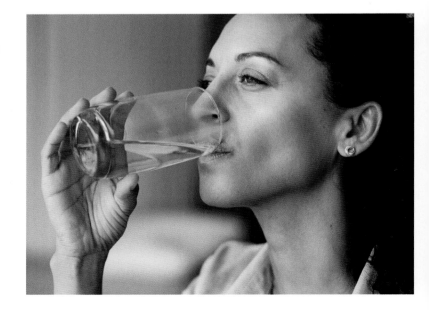

Hydrate with water

Water regulates body temperature, carries nutrients, removes waste products, and lubricates your joints – even low levels of dehydration can have a negative impact on both physical and mental wellbeing.

Balance and variety

By consuming a wide variety from the four food groups shown below you will be eating enough of the essential nutrients to maintain a good level of health. In some circumstances, when individual nutritional demand is increased, after injury or illness for example, nutrient supplementation may be beneficial. Ideally, talk to a nutrition healthcare professional to find out which supplements will be safe and appropriate.

FATS AND OILS

Prioritize oily fish, avocados, nuts, seeds, and their oils as your main sources of essential fatty acids. They also provide vitamin E, and the minerals selenium, magnesium, and zinc. Limit saturated fats as they are associated with an increased risk of cardiovascular disease. Trans fats – produced when unsaturated fats are hydrogenated – should be avoided.

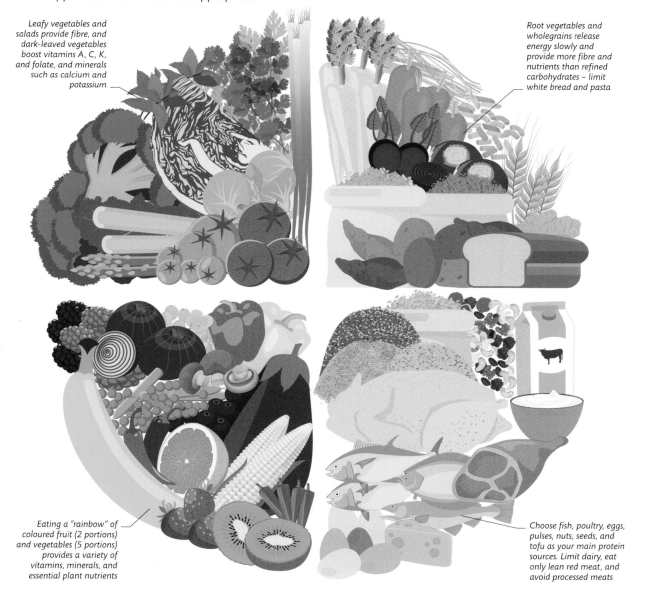

Leafy vegetables and salads provide fibre, and dark-leaved vegetables boost vitamins A, C, K, and folate, and minerals such as calcium and potassium

Root vegetables and wholegrains release energy slowly and provide more fibre and nutrients than refined carbohydrates – limit white bread and pasta

Eating a "rainbow" of coloured fruit (2 portions) and vegetables (5 portions) provides a variety of vitamins, minerals, and essential plant nutrients

Choose fish, poultry, eggs, pulses, nuts, seeds, and tofu as your main protein sources. Limit dairy, eat only lean red meat, and avoid processed meats

Adapting your diet

Sometimes it is necessary to adapt your diet to manage a condition such as excess weight gain, or to improve your health. To achieve this you may need to adjust quantities and ratios of the food groups, reduce your calorie intake, and/or make healthier food choices.

Why change your diet?

There are many benefits of changing your diet. Not only can it bring about increased energy levels, and improved digestion, mood, and quality of sleep, but it can also reduce the risks of conditions such as obesity, osteoarthritis, cardiovascular diseases, cancers, and type 2 diabetes. But adjusting the balance of nutrient groups is not always straightforward. For example, lowering blood cholesterol is not as simple as avoiding fats. There are different types of cholesterol; the potentially damaging very-low- and low-density lipoprotein (VLDL and LDL), and the beneficial high-density lipoprotein (HDL). Your body needs cholesterol, but it is the HDL to LDL ratio that is important as HDL helps to remove LDL from the blood. By increasing your intake of beneficial fats and reducing animal fats, you can help increase HDL and lower LDL.

WEIGHT MANAGEMENT

To lose weight, your energy intake must be less than your energy expenditure. To help achieve this, reduce your calorie intake and increase consumption of nutrient-dense foods (see below). Adjust your portion sizes, consume fewer refined carbohydrates and less saturated fat (see opposite). In addition, your exercise level and its intensity may need to be increased (see pp.152–55).

Worldwide, more than 39% of adults are overweight and 13% are obese

Energy and nutrient density

Energy provided by foods is most commonly reported in calories (kcal). Your calorie requirements are calculated on physical activity levels and your basal metabolic rate – the energy needed for basic functions, such as breathing and maintaining a heartbeat. Adult males require around 2,500 kcal and females 2,000 kcal per day, from a healthy balanced diet of food and drinks, but this also varies with age.

Nutrient density can vary

Look at the nutritional quality of your foods, not just the number of calories. Choose foods that are dense in nutrients rather than energy, to get the best quality and balance for your needs. These plates show how different foods can vary in their calorie content (energy density) and nutrient density.

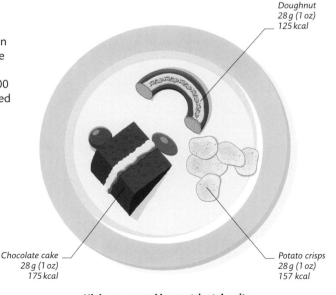

Doughnut
28 g (1 oz)
125 kcal

Chocolate cake
28 g (1 oz)
175 kcal

Potato crisps
28 g (1 oz)
157 kcal

High energy and low nutrient density

Change	Health benefits	Foods to eat	Foods to reduce or avoid
• Reducing saturated fat	• Reduces total blood cholesterol, and LDL • Reduces risk of cardiovascular diseases • Helps weight management • Improves mental health and cognitive function	• Steamed or boiled foods • Essential fatty acid omega-3 rich foods, such as oily fish, nuts, seeds, and avocados • Plant-based protein foods like pulses, soya, quinoa	• Fried or roasted foods • Fatty red meats • Processed meats • Cakes, pastries, and chocolate • High-fat dairy products such as hard cheese, cream, ghee, butter • Limit low-fat dairy products to a small yogurt or glass of milk or matchbox-sized piece of cheese
• Reducing salt	• Lowers blood pressure • Reduces risk of cardiovascular diseases	• Home-made fresh foods; make your own stocks, sauces, and gravies • Flavour foods with pepper, herbs, and spices instead of using salt • Choose snacks or canned foods with no added salt	• Ready-prepared meals • Processed and cured meats such as ham, sausages, bacon, salami • Salty snacks like crisps and nuts • Foods with added salt – check labels as these can include less obvious products like bread and cereals
• Reducing refined carbohydrates, or "free" sugars	• Helps weight management • Helps energy and mood balance • Reduces risk of type 2 diabetes • Improves digestion and dental health • Improves immune health	• High-fibre foods, such as fresh vegetables and fruit • Wholegrain and wholemeal varieties of bread and pasta • Alternative grains, such as quinoa, brown rice, spelt, rye, buckwheat, or oats	• High-sugar foods such as cakes, biscuits, pastries, and sweets • White breads and pasta • Foods with added sugar • Sugar-sweetened drinks (they also contain few nutrients), and limit fruit juice and alcohol

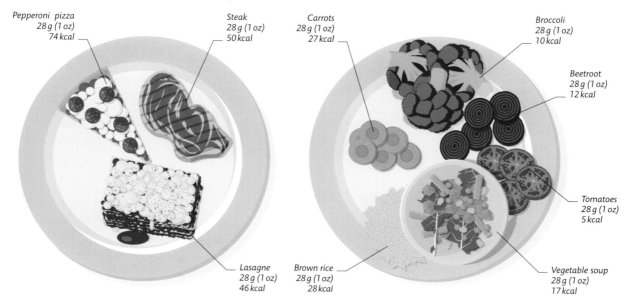

Pepperoni pizza
28 g (1 oz)
74 kcal

Steak
28 g (1 oz)
50 kcal

Lasagne
28 g (1 oz)
46 kcal

Carrots
28 g (1 oz)
27 kcal

Broccoli
28 g (1 oz)
10 kcal

Beetroot
28 g (1 oz)
12 kcal

Tomatoes
28 g (1 oz)
5 kcal

Brown rice
28 g (1 oz)
28 kcal

Vegetable soup
28 g (1 oz)
17 kcal

Medium energy and medium nutrient density

Low energy and high nutrient density

Alcohol, tobacco, and drugs

Learning about the effects alcohol, tobacco, and drugs can have on the body can help you make healthier life choices. Each one carries its own risks, and all can have a detrimental effect, not only on your physical health, but also on your mental wellbeing.

About alcohol

Alcohol is the most commonly used addictive substance. While light to moderate drinking may have some benefits, they are relatively small, and do not apply to everyone. It is recommended that you limit your intake to no more than 14 units (see below) per week, ideally less, spread over at least three days, and that you have several alcohol-free days per week. If you do not drink alcohol, do not start just because you think there might be health benefits.

In the short term, excessive alcohol use impairs judgement and causes accidents that can result in injury and complications such as pneumonia from aspiration of vomit. In the long term, heavy use can result in numerous detrimental effects on both mental and physical health, from depression, alcohol dependence, and addiction to liver failure, cardiovascular disease, brain damage, dementia, and many cancers.

 Worldwide, **13.5 per cent** of the **deaths** in the **20–39 age group are related to alcohol use**

WHAT IS A DRINK?

Guidelines as to what constitutes a standard drink vary from one country to another, typically ranging from 8 g (0.35 fl oz) of alcohol in the UK to 14 g (0.6 fl oz) in the US. Although all the drinks shown here contain 14 g (0.6 fl oz) of alcohol, they vary considerably in their calorie content (see p.148). Alcohol has almost as many calories as pure fat. Alcoholic drinks also contain sugars, which add to their calorie count and contribute to weight gain.

Wine can be up to 18% alcohol by volume

Alcohol and calorie content depend on the ratio of alcohol to mixer

Many of the calories in beer come from unfermented sugars

SPIRITS
44 ml (1.5 fl oz)
40% alcohol
95 calories

WINE
150 ml (5 fl oz)
12% alcohol
125 calories

SPIRITS AND MIXER
192ml (6.5 fl oz)
5% alcohol
150 calories

BEER
355 ml (12 fl oz)
5% alcohol
155 calories

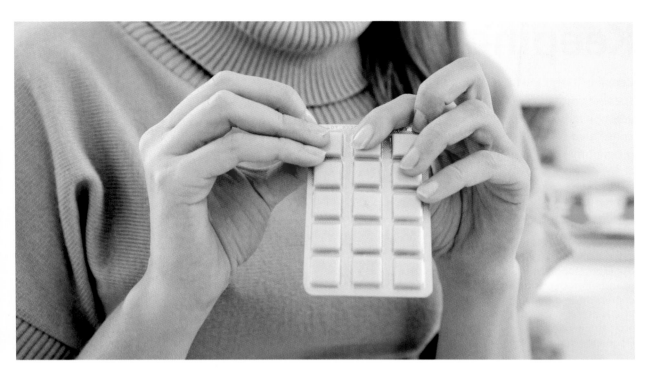

Tobacco use

Whether you smoke it or chew it, tobacco is not only addictive, but it also increases your risk of developing serious health problems, including many cancers. Smoking can also reduce fertility, prematurely age your skin, and harm the health of those around you. Giving up tobacco can be difficult, but the good news is that after only one year of not smoking, your risk is reduced by half. To make it easier to quit:

- Your doctor can prescribe medication that reduces withdrawal symptoms and eases cravings.
- Join a support group and/or find a "quit buddy" who wants to stop, and ask your friends and family to help you.

Risks associated with drugs

The effects of drugs vary considerably, depending on the substance. But repeated use of many can lead to addiction that not only has a negative impact on relationships and daily life, but also results in painful withdrawal symptoms when a person stops using them. Long-term use of any drug can leave you susceptible to serious health problems, ranging from cardiovascular disease to blood-borne infections, and is linked to severe mental-health issues. But with the right help it is possible to be drug free; start by talking to your family doctor or local drug clinic.

Nicotine-replacement therapy

The addictive substance in cigarettes is nicotine. If used correctly, chewing nicotine gum (or wearing patches) provides your body with enough nicotine to reduce the withdrawal symptoms experienced when you stop smoking.

ELECTRONIC CIGARETTES

Also known as e-cigarettes, these are battery-powered devices that mimic the effect of smoking. The user inhales the nicotine as a vapour ("vaping") instead of breathing in the toxic tar and carbon monoxide from burning tobacco. There is evidence that e-cigarettes can help people to give up smoking, although the effects of long-term use – possibly including nicotine addiction – are not clear.

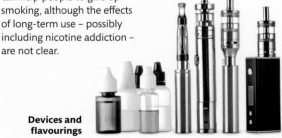

Devices and flavourings

Keeping fit

Keeping fit begins with reducing sitting time and spending more time being active. Any activity that gets you moving and using your muscles can be considered exercise. Before starting a training programme, get the green light from your doctor.

Exercise

Regular exercise has a profoundly positive impact on physical and mental wellbeing. It can improve weight control, improve sleep quality, and reduce stress. Exercise may also reduce the risk of chronic ailments, such as joint and back pain, cardiovascular disease, type 2 diabetes, depression, and dementia.

It is useful to structure your exercise programme using the following principles: Frequency, Intensity, Time, Type, and Rate of progression (FITTR). Adults should be active up to five days per week, alternating exercises to allow muscle groups to rest. Aim for at least 150 minutes of moderate or 75 minutes of vigorous activity or a combination of both each week. Progress in small increments to avoid injury.

Benefits of exercise
Regular exercise benefits many parts of the body, making it function more efficiently.

Brain and mental wellbeing
Exercise increases the delivery of blood, oxygen, and nutrients to the brain

Heart
The heart becomes stronger and it distributes blood more efficiently

Lungs
Exercise increases lung capacity

Liver
Metabolic rate is improved

Bones and joints
Exercise strengthens your bones and joints

Muscles
Strong muscles improve your posture and flexibility

Circulation
Arteries widen, increasing blood flow to the muscles

TIPS FOR SUSTAINING AN EXERCISE PROGRAMME

- Understand the benefits of exercise and the programme you are following.
- Practise exercises or sports that you enjoy.
- Set achievable goals.
- Be efficient and build exercise or physical activity into your daily routine.
- Be consistent – small increments each week lead to big improvements in the long run.

- Monitor your progress. Wear a fitness tracker or keep a diary of goals achieved.
- Rest for 24-48 hours to reduce your risk of injury. Remember, you can rest some muscle groups while exercising others.
- A healthy diet is essential (see pp.146–47).
- Challenge your friends and encourage each other.
- Seek professional advice when necessary.

Strengthen your muscles and bones

Resistance training improves muscle strength, which is necessary for all activities, helps build and maintain strong bones, and also assists in the control of blood pressure, blood glucose, and body weight. It can be performed at home or at the gym two days per week and may include lifting weights, using resistance bands, push-ups, sit-ups, or even gardening. Aim to work hard enough so that another repetition of the activity would be difficult to complete.

Maintaining flexibility

Activities that improve balance, flexibility, and agility include yoga, Pilates, Tai Chi, and stretching, and should be done on at least two days a week. These are complex activities requiring controlled coordination of numerous muscles groups, which help develop postural stability and, in older adults, help reduce the risk of falls (see p.156). These types of activity are also ideal activities for mental rest and reflection.

Exercise for cardiovascular health

Activities that improve endurance and cardiovascular fitness include walking, running, cycling, swimming, climbing stairs, and participating in sports. Moderate activity increases your heart and respiratory rate, but you're able to talk, and you will have a light sweat after 10 minutes. Vigorous activity raises your heart rate, makes you breathe hard and fast, you cannot say more than a few words without pausing, and you sweat after a few minutes.

Healthy heart and lungs
Swimming and cycling are good exercises for fitness and endurance without placing impact stress on the joints. Taking time to warm up and cool down may reduce strain on the muscles in the shoulders, back, and thighs.

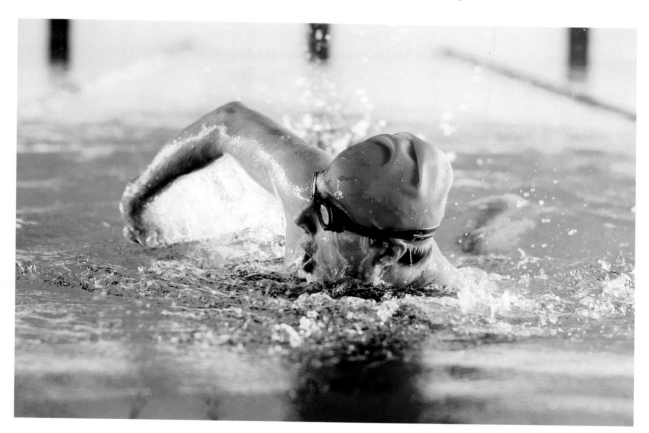

Exercise for special groups

Appropriate physical activity will greatly benefit people suffering from a health condition or who are getting older. However, such groups require a specifically targeted and supervised training programme.

MONITORING YOUR ACTIVITIES

Wearable devices have become highly sophisticated tools for tracking health metrics, such as heart rate, physical activity, sleep patterns, and calorie intake. These devices provide useful information for monitoring improvements in your health and the body's response to exercise.

When can I exercise?

Remaining active and preserving health becomes increasingly important with age or in the context of chronic conditions, where immense physical and mental health benefits may be achieved. For example, exercise may preserve the cardiac function in patients with cardiovascular disease such as angina, resistance training helps maintain bone mass and manage osteoporosis, and stretching and agility exercises maintain range of motion and improve joint function in people with arthritis. In these scenarios, exercise programmes must be individualized. Appropriate professional advice, supervision, and monitoring can improve success and safety.

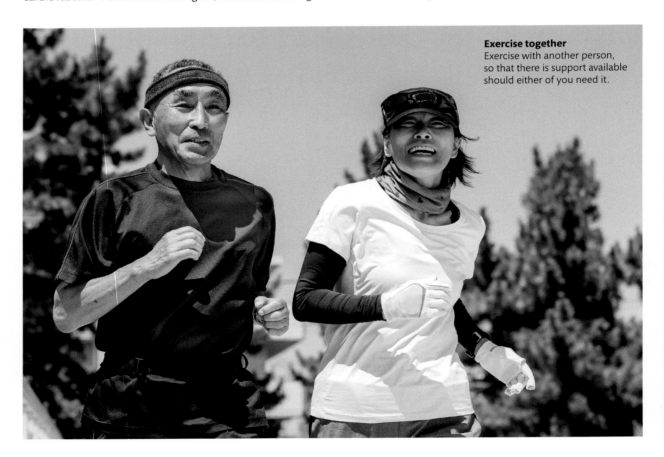

Exercise together
Exercise with another person, so that there is support available should either of you need it.

Know your limits

Exercise frequency, intensity, time, type, and rate of progression (FITTR, see p.152) will depend on the individual's baseline ability. Clinical evaluation and exercise testing prior to starting an exercise or rehabilitation programme are essential and provide insight into the level at which exercise can be initiated safely. Consideration is also given to factors, such as medication or pacemakers, that may influence the body's response to exercise. Two useful metrics to monitor intensity include your current heart rate as a percentage of your maximum heart rate, and rate of perceived exertion.

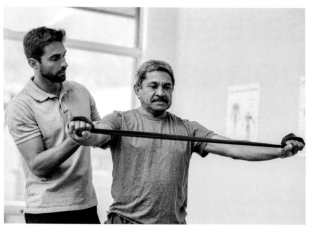

Your maximum heart rate can be calculated by subtracting your age from 220

Training under supervision
A training plan devised by a professional, such as a physiotherapist, will ensure that you do the exercises that are right for you and that you do them in the correct way.

SPECIAL CONSIDERATION

Seek medical advice before starting any exercise programme to ensure that you do exercises that are safe and most beneficial.

Stop the activity and seek help immediately if you feel dizzy, feel ill, or experience any pain, including muscular or chest pain.

Chronic illness	Special considerations	Good exercises to consider
Diabetes	• Monitor blood glucose levels to prevent hypoglycaemia. • Keep hydrated. • Monitor heart rate and blood pressure. • Pay extra attention to foot care and ulcer prevention. • Exercise with a partner.	• Resistance training • Aerobic exercises
Cardiovascular disease	• Some medication (such as beta blockers) or pacemakers may influence your heart rate during exercise. • Exercise under supervision and stop activity if symptoms occur.	• Moderate intensity cardiovascular exercise and resistance training
Obesity	• To lose weight, exercise should be combined with dietary changes. • Take extra care to prevent injuries.	• Focus on aerobic activities
Osteoporosis	• Take extra care to prevent falls.	• Pilates, Tai Chi • Weight-bearing and resistance exercises
Arthritis	• Reduce repetitive joint impact. • Use appropriate equipment, e.g. well-cushioned, shock-absorbing shoes. • Adequate warm-up and cool-down can minimize pain.	• Prioritize exercises that encourage joint range of motion • Low impact activities such as walking, swimming, or cycling • Include functional activities, such as sit-to-stand and step-ups
Cancer	• Start with light intensity exercise for short durations. • Modify exercise type and intensity around the time of treatment. • Avoid physical inactivity. • Bone metastases may require reduction of impact activities.	• Depends on type of cancer and treatment • Team sports (e.g. cycling or bowls)

Safeguarding your bones and muscles

Bones and muscles are dynamic tissues that remodel continuously to accommodate for the forces they endure. The potential size and strength of bone and muscle tissue is determined by genetics. However, you can take steps yourself to maintain and strengthen your bones and muscles, such as following a healthy diet and taking regular exercise.

Healthy bones

Bone mass declines steadily with age. Post-menopausal women may also lose bone mass due to hormonal changes. Osteoporosis occurs when bone mass decreases to the level at which fractures can occur without significant trauma. To maintain optimum bone mass it is important to:

- Be active
- Get enough protein, calcium, and vitamin D in your diet
- Maintain a healthy BMI (see pp.24–25)
- Avoid smoking
- Reduce your alcohol intake
- Maintain your balance, agility, and coordination to prevent falls (see below)

Decreasing bone mass

This chart shows how bone mass (related to the amount of calcium stored in the bones) naturally decreases with age. Changes may not be apparent in your daily life, so seek advice from your doctor regarding your osteoporosis risk.

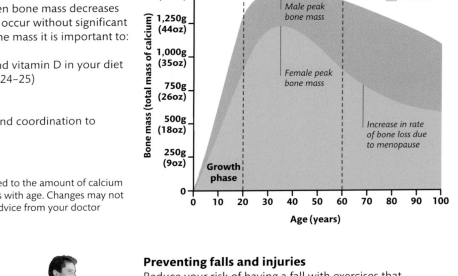

KEY
- Male
- Female

Male peak bone mass

Female peak bone mass

Increase in rate of bone loss due to menopause

Growth phase

Bone mass (total mass of calcium): 1,500g (53oz), 1,250g (44oz), 1,000g (35oz), 750g (26oz), 500g (18oz), 250g (9oz), 0

Age (years): 0, 10, 20, 30, 40, 50, 60, 70, 80, 90, 100

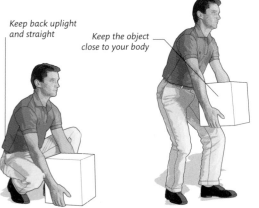

Keep back uplight and straight

Keep the object close to your body

Keep your back straight   **Lift with your legs**

Preventing falls and injuries

Reduce your risk of having a fall with exercises that build strength, balance, and agility, such as yoga or Tai Chi. Other steps you can take include avoiding or reducing alcohol consumption, having your sight tested, and getting any medication reviewed by your physician. Minimize hazards at home by removing clutter and exposed cables, use non-slip rugs for slippery surfaces, ensure that there is adequate lighting, mop up spillages immediately, and use appropriate footwear.

Right way to lift heavy objects

Prevent back strain when lifting heavy objects by using your leg muscles to lift the weight. Bend your knees and keep the back straight when lifting, and try to make the lift a smooth movement.

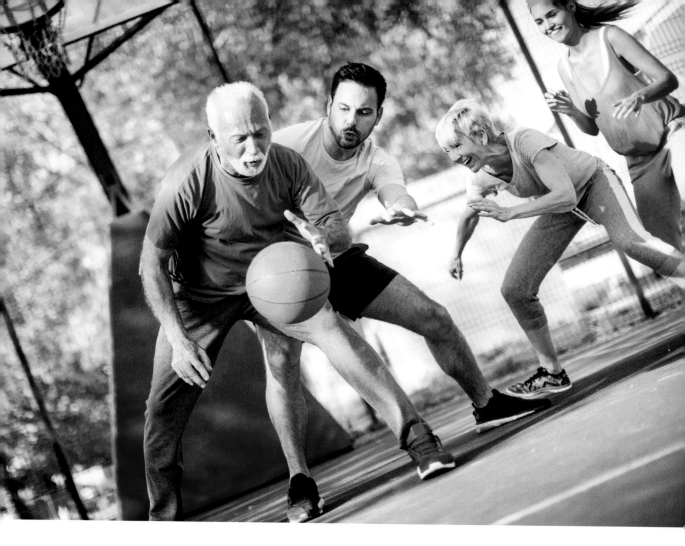

Strengthening exercises

Weight-bearing exercises, with appropriate impact, and muscle-strengthening exercises maintain strong bones and stimulate muscle growth. On most days, healthy adults should include 20–30 minutes of moderate impact activity – people with osteoporosis should spend 20 minutes on lower impact exercises. Prolonged sitting should be avoided. For guidance:

- Low impact – walking, stair climbing.
- Moderate impact – dancing, jogging, running, team and racket sports, skipping.
- High impact – basketball, star jumps, track events.

Strengthening muscles requires movement against resistance, such as exercises with free weights, resistance bands, or using body weight. Remember to warm up, stretch, and gradually build up strength to avoid injury.

Appropriate impact

Basketball can place a lot of stress on the bones and joints, so care should be taken when playing. However, it is good exercise to help maintain coordination, agility, and balance.

Healthy diet

As part of a healthy, balanced diet (see pp.146–47), adequate protein, calcium, and vitamin D intake are essential for strong bones and muscles. Adults require at least 700mg (¾₂₅oz) of calcium every day. Older adults and breastfeeding women require up to 1.25g (½₂₅oz) of calcium per day. Vitamin D helps the body absorb and utilise calcium effectively, and can be obtained through safe sun exposure (10–30 minutes per day), dietary sources (such as oily fish, eggs, and fortified cereals), or taking supplements.

Keeping your skin healthy

Your skin performs a wide range of different tasks for your body, from helping to maintain body temperature to making vitamin D – vital for bone health – when exposed to the sun.

Day-to-day skin health

Everything you do, from eating and drinking to sleep and stress, can affect your skin. A good balanced diet that includes fruit, vegetables, and foods with natural oils (see pp.146–49) helps keep skin healthy. Drinking plenty of fluids keeps it hydrated, and avoiding alcohol, or sticking to the recommended limits, can prevent dehydration. Manage your weight, but avoid crash diets as repeatedly losing and regaining weight can take its toll on your skin. Do not smoke (or quit if you do) – it prematurely ages skin by damaging the collagen that provides elasticity and strength.

Learn to manage stress (see p.165) as uncontrolled stress can trigger conditions such as eczema. Poor sleep is another trigger. However, a good night's sleep (see p.165) boosts blood flow to the skin, aiding repair and regeneration.

Wash daily to prevent skin infections, but avoid strong soap products as these can disrupt the balance of natural oils in your skin. If you have very dry skin, you can use emollients as a soap substitute. Use daily moisturizer with UV protection. Check your skin regularly and report any unusual coloration or marks to your doctor (see pp.98–99).

Preventing infection

Areas of skin-to-skin contact where the environment is warm and moist, such as in the groin or underarms, can be susceptible to fungal infections, so ensure you dry them carefully after washing. Keep areas of damaged skin, such as bites or scratches, clean and, if necessary, covered to prevent bacterial infections from developing.

FOOT-CARE ESSENTIALS

- Check your feet for sore patches, redness, or numbness at least once a week – or more often if you have diabetes or circulatory problems.
- Keep your feet cool and dry – fungal foot infections like athlete's foot thrive in warm, moist environments. Dry feet thoroughly after washing.
- In hot weather, wear open, well-ventilated footwear made from non-synthetic and breathable materials.
- Change your shoes regularly – always after sports activities – and wear absorbent, cotton socks.
- Apply moisturizer to dry skin, especially around the heels, to prevent cracked skin.
- Warts and veruccas (see p.99) are caused by the human papillomavirus (HPV), and spread by skin-to-skin contact and contact with contaminated surfaces, so wear flip-flops in communal bathing areas and avoid sharing footwear or towels.

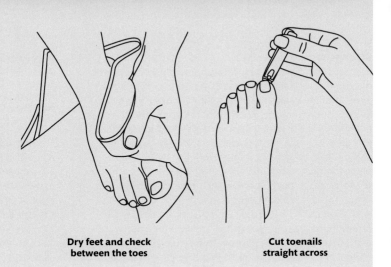

Dry feet and check between the toes

Cut toenails straight across

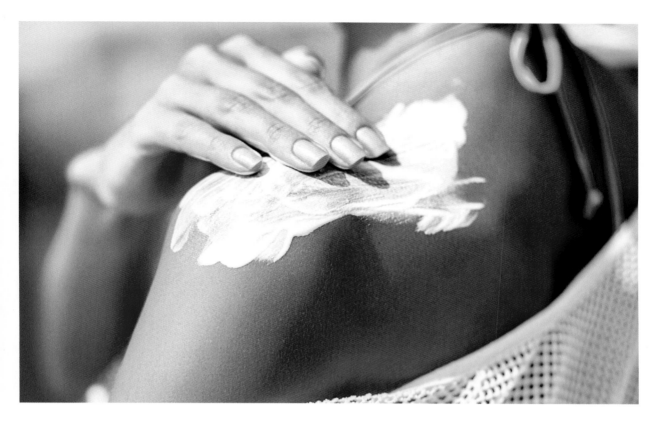

Use a strong sunscreen
Apply plenty of sunscreen with sun protection factor (SPF) 30 (50 for very pale skin) and good UVA protection 30 minutes before you go out. Reapply every two hours, or right after swimming.

Protect skin from ultraviolet light
Ultraviolet (UV) radiation from sun rays (or tanning beds and sunlamps) damages the skin and is the main cause of skin ageing and skin cancer (see pp.98–99). It is important to protect your skin to reduce the risk of skin damage.
- Apply a strong sunscreen – but remember it is only a filter; it does not block all the rays. You can get sunburn from indirect rays as well as direct sunlight.
- Cover your skin and wear UV-blocking sunglasses.
- Stay in the shade, especially between 11 am and 3 pm when the sun is at its highest.
- Do not use tanning beds and sunlamps.

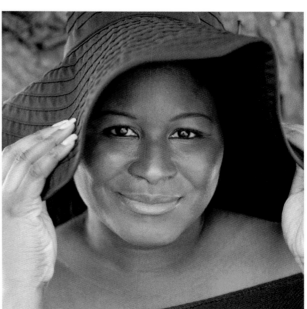

Wear a wide-brimmed hat
Choose a hat with at least a 5–7.5 cm (2–3 in) brim because it offers better protection to areas often exposed to intense sun, such as the scalp, ears, eyes, forehead, and nose.

Ear health

Maintaining good general health through diet and fitness can minimize the risk of conditions that can lead to hearing problems and reduce the likelihood of age-related hearing loss. However, exposure to loud noises can damage your inner ear and lead to irreversible hearing loss.

Protect your hearing

More than half of the cases of hearing loss are preventable. Make sure your vaccinations are up to date (see pp.144–45), as many infections can cause hearing problems. Keep your ears clean and dry to prevent infections; wear ear plugs when swimming, or in the shower if necessary.

Be mindful of the level of noise in your surroundings. Resist the temptation to increase the volume on your headphones, speakers, or television. Wear ear defenders if you work in a noisy environment or use loud equipment like drills for DIY at home. Professional musicians can use vented ear plugs that allow a controlled level of sound in, while also protecting their ears.

🔊))) **More than 1 billion young people globally risk developing hearing loss through exposure to loud music**

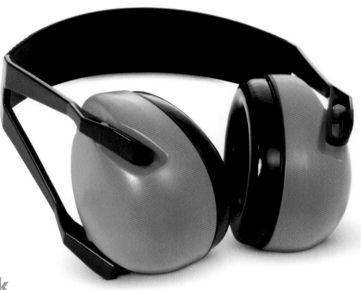

Ear defenders
These are designed to protect your hearing from hazardous noise pollution, especially in the workplace. They each carry a rating that indicates the level of protection offered.

Reusable ear plugs
Use these to protect your ears in water, or even to aid sleep. Clean your ear plugs regularly to minimize the risk of developing an ear infection.

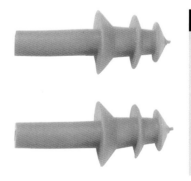

CLEANING YOUR EARS

The ear canal (see p.110) is protected by ear wax, but too little or too much can cause ear infections. Wipe your outer ear with a washcloth and warm water, but the ear canal is self-cleaning, so never put anything, especially not a cotton bud, inside it as you can push wax further in, or even damage the eardrum. If you have a build-up of wax, a few drops of olive oil twice a day for a few days will soften it and it should fall out. Over-the-counter eardrops made to loosen earwax are also available. Consult your doctor if this does not help.

Eye health

A nutritious, balanced diet packed with colourful fruits and leafy green vegetables, rich in vitamins and minerals (see pp.146–47), and adequate sleep are essential for eye health. Have regular eye check-ups (pp.102–109) to detect any vision problems, and because signs of some underlying health problems can be seen in your eyes.

Look after your eyes

- Maintain good hygiene to prevent infection. Wipe around your eyes with cotton wool and warm water, using a separate pad for each eye. Remove all your eye make-up before you go to bed.
- Quit smoking and limit your alcohol intake as both are known to increase the risk of eye disease.
- Wear sunglasses in bright sun. Wraparound sunglasses are useful if you are susceptible to hayfever, and dark goggles are essential in the snow, even on a dull day.
- If you are doing any DIY or work in an environment where there is dust or chemicals, always wear goggles. Never touch your eyes after working with harmful products.
- When working at a computer screen, take a break every 20 minutes and look at an object at least 6 m (20 ft) away for at least 20 seconds.

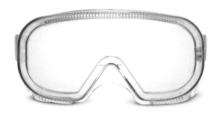

Wraparound safety goggles
Wear these if there is a risk of dust, particles, or chemicals entering your eyes. Make sure they fit securely before you start.

Sunglasses make a difference
UV radiation from the sun's rays (or a tanning bed) can cause a variety of eye conditions, including cataracts. Choose good-quality dark glasses with a safe level of UV protection; ideally wear a wide-brimmed hat, too.

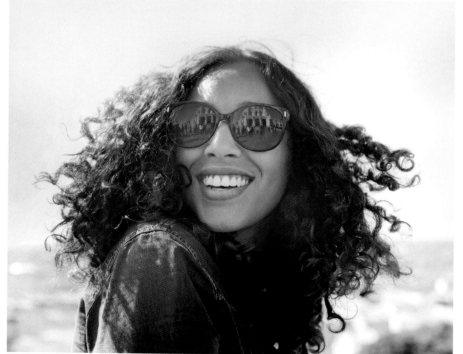

Vitamins A and C help to preserve good eyesight

Sexual health

Sex is an important part of life, affecting your physical, mental, emotional, and social wellbeing. Being in good sexual health also means staying safe by being well-informed, careful, and respectful to both yourself and others.

Practise safer sex
Of paramount importance in good sexual health is making an effort to prevent unintended pregnancies, as well as avoiding sexually transmitted infections (STIs) – and seeking care and treatment promptly if they do develop. There is a wide range of contraceptives available to prevent pregnancy; the choice largely depends on your medical history and your lifestyle. Alcohol and drug use can reduce inhibitions and impair judgement, so avoiding them reduces the chances of engaging in risky behaviour. The most effective way to avoid an STI is to use a condom (male or female), too, and to limit the number of sexual partners. When used correctly, condoms prevent the transmission

Making the most of your sex life
Talking, and more importantly, listening, to each other about your feelings, preferences, and desires, can bring you closer together and make sex more fulfilling.

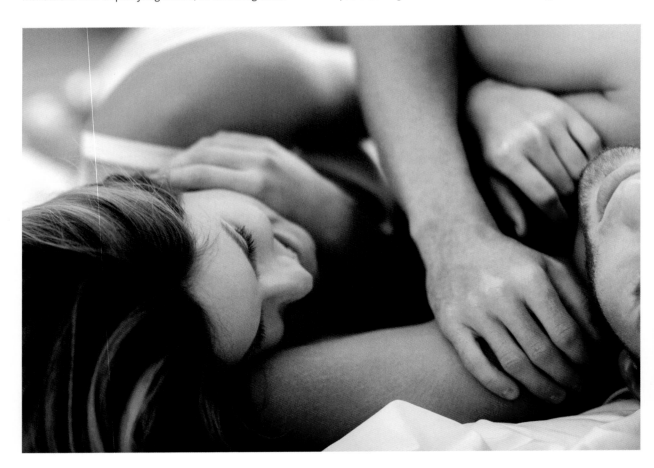

of STIs, such as HIV, chlamydia, and gonorrhoea, that are spread by genital fluids. They can reduce the risk of infections that are spread by skin-to-skin contact, like genital herpes, syphilis, and human papillomavirus, only if the condom covers the infected area. If you are using condoms, avoid oil-based moisturizers and petroleum jelly as they can damage them, or cause them to tear – it is safer to use water-based lubricants.

Regular screening is important

Some people experience symptoms of STIs, such as unusual discharge or bleeding, sores, rashes, or itching, but many have no symptoms, so if you are changing partners or have multiple partners, it is a good idea to have regular screening. See your doctor or visit a sexual health clinic prior to initiating sexual contact with a new partner; if your protection was inadequate: for example, a condom split; or you suspect your partner might have an STI. Prompt diagnosis and treatment is essential as some infections can cause cancers or spread into the pelvis, causing inflammation that can lead to infertility. If you are diagnosed with an infection, it is important to tell current or previous sexual partners.

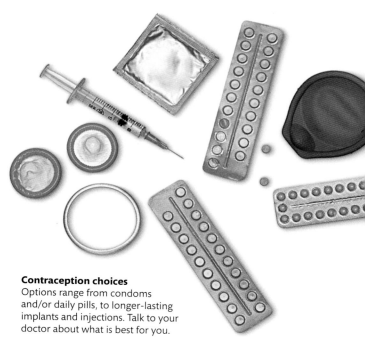

Contraception choices
Options range from condoms and/or daily pills, to longer-lasting implants and injections. Talk to your doctor about what is best for you.

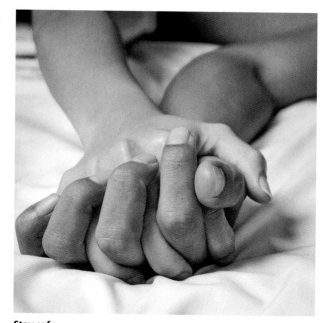

Stay safe
Enjoy your sexuality in a way you are comfortable with. If either of you has been diagnosed with an STI, then avoid penetrative sex until your treatment has been completed.

It is estimated that between **6 and 9 billion condoms** are sold every year

MAXIMIZING FERTILITY

Maintaining good health through diet (see pp.146–49) and exercise (see pp.152–55) is a key way to maximize fertility. Being overweight or underweight can also affect ovulation – the optimal body mass index (BMI) for conception is between 20 and 25 (see pp.24–25). Smoking has been shown to reduce fertility in females and has been linked to poor semen quality. Women planning to conceive are advised to avoid alcohol as it not only affects fertility, but it also poses a risk to the unborn child. Men should not exceed the recommended daily maximum alcohol intake as excessive amounts can affect sperm quality – hot baths have been found to affect male fertility, too. Likewise, recreational drug use should be avoided.

Psychological health

Maintaining a healthy mental state is as important as maintaining physical health. If you struggle with physical health problems, you are more at risk of mental health issues; likewise, inability to deal with stress and anxiety can increase your susceptibility to illness.

Live life well
Scientific research shows that there is a strong mind-body connection – how you think affects how you feel, which in turn affects how you behave. Psychological health is affected by numerous factors, many of which you control. Exercise and a healthy diet (see pp.146–49 and 152–55) contribute to mental wellbeing, as will learning to manage stress and making sure you have enough good-quality sleep. Social factors, or how well and how much you connect with others, can also play a significant role. Conversely, smoking and alcohol or drug consumption have a negative impact (see pp.150–51).

Promoting positive emotions
We are all intrinsically motivated to seek happiness. This psychological model defines the five elements essential to your wellbeing. By gaining an understanding of each one and taking steps to pursue them in your thoughts and actions, you can enhance your resilience, which also helps protect you from stress and anxiety.

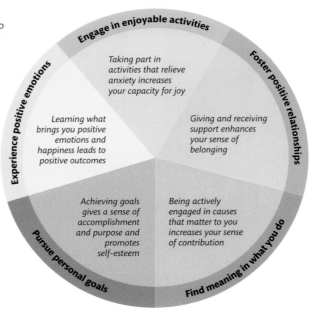

Engage in enjoyable activities
Taking part in activities that relieve anxiety increases your capacity for joy

Foster positive relationships
Giving and receiving support enhances your sense of belonging

Find meaning in what you do
Being actively engaged in causes that matter to you increases your sense of contribution

Pursue personal goals
Achieving goals gives a sense of accomplishment and purpose and promotes self-esteem

Experience positive emotions
Learning what brings you positive emotions and happiness leads to positive outcomes

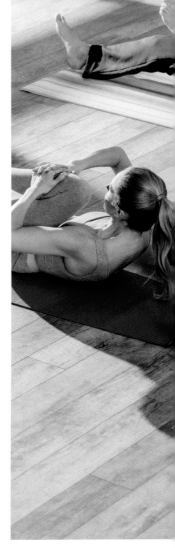

Making social connections
Humans are social animals with a natural desire to connect to others. Taking part in physical activity classes not only improves physical health, enhances mood and confidence, and gives you a sense of accomplishment, but also provides you with a source of company.

30 minutes of low-intensity aerobic exercise daily helps positive mood

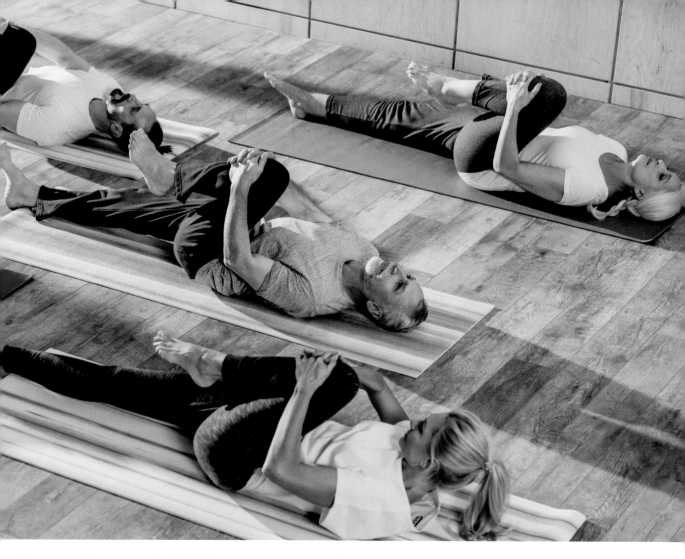

Ensure you have a good night's sleep

The body needs around seven hours of sleep a night in order to repair, rest, and recover from the day – without it, it is difficult to cope with everyday stress. If you do not sleep well, try making a few changes:

- Make your bedroom a calm, relaxing place to be and leave TVs, phones, and tablets outside the room – the "blue" light stimulates the brain, preventing sleep.
- Having a bedtime routine can stimulate the sleep hormone melatonin, enhancing your chances of sleeping well; set your alarm to wake up at a regular time.
- Eat your last meal 2 to 3 hours before bedtime, so that your body can digest the food before you fall asleep.
- Avoid exercising within four hours of bedtime as this stimulates the stress hormone cortisol, preventing sleep.
- Wear an eye mask to shut out any distracting light.

Learn to manage stress

Under stress the brain releases the stress hormone cortisol. Over time, high levels of this hormone can raise blood pressure, disrupt sleep, and seriously affect your mental health. Try a few of the following tips to reduce the levels.

- Exercising regularly can relieve mental stress and anxiety.
- Find a support network, friend, or family member to confide in; talking about feelings can reduce anxiety.
- Consider which specific situations or people increase your stress levels, so you can avoid, anticipate, or learn to manage them better.
- Restrict time on social media; comparing your real life to the "curated" ideal life of others can lead to depression.
- Use breathing exercises to help you relax. When you are feeling anxious, stop, sit down, and breathe in for a count of 4 and out for a count of 8; repeat until relaxed.

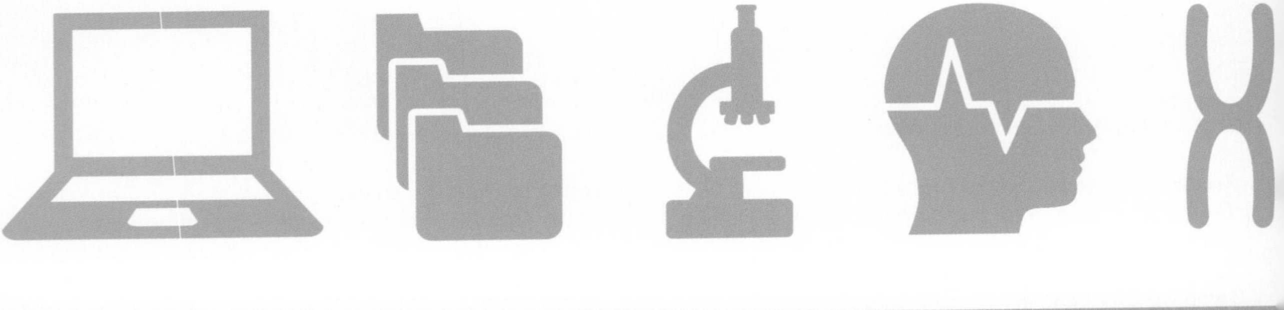

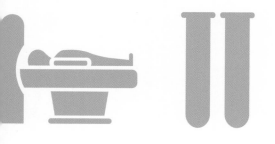

Other tests and your records

Other medical tests

There are a large number of medical tests that can be used to assess your health, screen for early indications of disease, or diagnose disorders after symptoms have appeared. The following pages outline some of the more common procedures used primarily for diagnosis.

Chest scan
This colour-enhanced MRI scan of the chest shows the heart (large red area in the centre) and blood vessels in a healthy man.

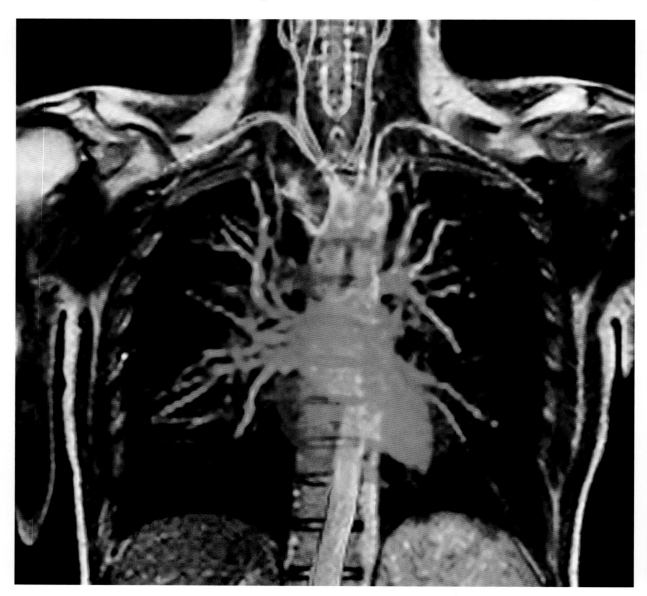

CARDIOVASCULAR AND RESPIRATORY SYSTEM TESTS

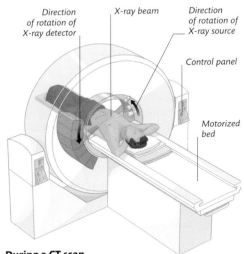

Direction of rotation of X-ray detector

X-ray beam

Direction of rotation of X-ray source

Control panel

Motorized bed

During a CT scan
You lie on a table that moves you into the scanner. The X-ray source and detector rotate around you as the scan is performed.

Chest CT scan
A CT (computed tomography) scan is an image made using X-rays passed through the body at different angles. A computer processes the X-ray information to create a cross-sectional image of internal structures. Sometimes, a special substance (a contrast material) may first be injected to make tissues more clearly visible. Chest CT scans may be carried out to investigate tumours, narrowed or blocked airways, or structural problems in your heart or nearby blood vessels.

Chest MRI scan
In MRI (magnetic resonance imaging), a strong magnetic field stimulates your cells to emit radio signals, and a computer processes the signals to create detailed images of body structures. In some cases, a contrast medium may be used to make tissues show up more clearly. A chest MRI may be used to investigate problems such as tumours, or abnormalities in your lungs, heart, blood vessels, or blood flow. For an MRI scan, you lie on a table inside a tunnel while the scan is being performed.

MRA
Angiography is used to image the blood vessels. MRA (magnetic resonance angiography) is a form of MRI (below, left). It is often carried out using a special substance (a contrast material) injected before the scan to make your blood vessels show up more clearly. However, sometimes it is performed without using a contrast medium. MRA is used to investigate problems that may be causing reduced blood flow, such as narrowed, blocked, or damaged arteries, or abnormal blood-vessel structures. A chest MRA may be used to look at the coronary arteries, aorta (the main artery from the heart), or pulmonary arteries (supplying blood to the lungs).

Carotid artery Doppler scan
This procedure is a special type of ultrasound scanning that uses very high-frequency sound waves to produce images of blood flow in the carotid arteries (the major arteries in the neck supplying blood to the brain). The images appear instantly and in real time, so your blood can be seen as it flows through the arteries. The technique can be used to investigate possible strokes by revealing any blockages, narrowed areas, or other problems that restrict blood flow to the brain.

Scanning the carotid arteries
Gel is applied to your neck, then a transducer is moved over your skin to scan the arteries. The procedure is quick and painless.

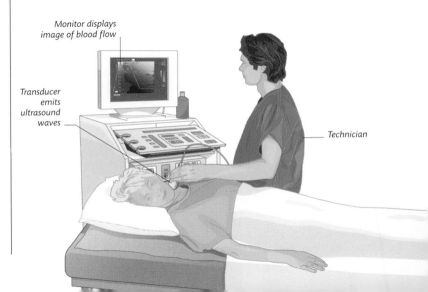

Monitor displays image of blood flow

Transducer emits ultrasound waves

Technician

Angiography

Angiography is X-ray imaging of the heart and blood vessels. It may be used to help detect problems such as a narrowed coronary artery or an aneurysm (a bulge in a weakened area of artery wall). A thin, flexible, hollow tube (catheter) is inserted into an artery at your groin or wrist and guided to the area to be examined. A contrast dye (a substance that blocks X-rays) is then injected through the catheter, so that the heart structure and blood vessels will show up clearly, and X-rays are taken as the dye flows through the structures.

Bronchoscopy

In this test, a thin, flexible viewing tube called a bronchoscope is inserted into your nose or mouth and guided down to the airways in your lungs. The tube has a light and a camera at its tip, which enables the doctor to view your airways directly, either through an eyepiece or on a monitor. Bronchoscopy can reveal problems such as inflammation or tumours. Instruments can be passed down the tube to remove foreign objects or take tissue samples (biopsies).

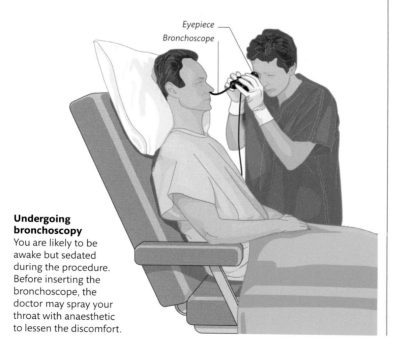

Eyepiece
Bronchoscope

Undergoing bronchoscopy
You are likely to be awake but sedated during the procedure. Before inserting the bronchoscope, the doctor may spray your throat with anaesthetic to lessen the discomfort.

BLOOD AND IMMUNE SYSTEM TESTS

Blood tests for allergy

If you develop signs of an allergic reaction, such as runny nose, itchy eyes, or a skin rash, the doctor may order a blood test to find the cause. In an allergic reaction, your immune system over-reacts and makes too much of a type of antibody known as immunoglobulin E (IgE). Testing a sample of your blood for the presence of IgE can reveal whether or not your symptoms are due to an allergy. Different varieties of IgE are produced in response to specific allergens, and if your symptoms are due to allergy, your blood may also be tested for allergen-specific varieties of IgE to pinpoint the precise substance that is causing the allergic reaction.

Exclusion diet testing for allergy

A food allergy or intolerance can cause symptoms such as bloating, abdominal pain, diarrhoea, nausea, vomiting, wheezing, sneezing, skin rash, and itchy eyes. Your doctor may advise a food elimination diet to find the specific food or foods responsible. This involves avoiding the suspect food or ingredient (such as a food additive) for two to six weeks to see if your symptoms improve, then reintroducing that food or substance to see if the symptoms return. If symptoms do diminish or disappear then reappear when the food is reintroduced, allergy or intolerance to that food is probably the cause. Your doctor may ask you to keep a food diary during this time to see how your symptoms progress. You should only follow an exclusion diet under medical supervision.

Tumour marker tests

Tumour markers are substances (most commonly proteins) that the body produces in response to cancer or that are produced by the cancer cells themselves. These markers can be found in blood, urine, other body fluids, faeces, and certain body tissues. Your doctor will take a sample of a body fluid (often blood) or tissue and send it to a laboratory for specialized testing to detect the presence and levels of tumour markers. Doctors may use tumour marker tests to help in diagnosing a cancer, and also to plan and monitor the progress of treatment.

DIGESTIVE AND ENDOCRINE SYSTEM TESTS

Digestive system MRI

MRI (magnetic resonance imaging) scans of the abdomen and pelvis use a strong magnetic field and radio waves to provide images of your digestive tract (mouth, throat, oesophagus, stomach, small intestine, and large intestine); digestive organs, such as the liver and pancreas; and other structures associated with the digestive system, such as blood vessels. A doctor may order an MRI scan of the digestive system to identify or assess problems such as tumours, narrowing or blockages in the digestive tract, or changes due to diseases such as cirrhosis of the liver, pancreatitis (inflammation of the pancreas), or inflammatory bowel disorders, such as Crohn's disease or ulcerative colitis. For some types of MRI scan, you may be asked to drink a substance (known as a contrast medium) before the scan so that particular structures will show up more clearly on the scan.

Faecal micoscopy

If you have severe diarrhoea due to food poisoning or a suspected digestive infection, your doctor may ask you to provide a sample of faeces for analysis. In the laboratory, a small amount of the faeces is examined under a microscope to look for parasites, such as worms, or for parasite eggs or larvae. The sample will also be examined to check for harmful bacteria, or to detect white blood cells, which can indicate infection.

Gastroscopy

In gastroscopy, a thin, flexible viewing instrument (called a gastroscope) is passed down your throat to view the oesophagus (gullet), stomach, and duodenum (the first

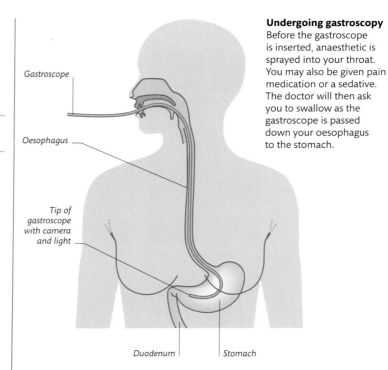

Gastroscope

Oesophagus

Tip of gastroscope with camera and light

Duodenum

Stomach

Undergoing gastroscopy
Before the gastroscope is inserted, anaesthetic is sprayed into your throat. You may also be given pain medication or a sedative. The doctor will then ask you to swallow as the gastroscope is passed down your oesophagus to the stomach.

part of the small intestine). The gastroscope has a light and a camera at the tip; the camera sends images to a monitor. Gastroscopy is used to investigate problems of the upper digestive tract, such as indigestion, difficulty swallowing, stomach ulcers, bleeding, or narrowing of the oesophagus. The gastrosope can also be used to take tissue samples, remove growths or foreign objects, or treat bleeding or narrowed areas.

Thyroid scanning

In a thyroid scan, you are given a small amount of a radioactive substance, usually iodine (which the thyroid gland easily absorbs), by injection or by mouth. You will have to wait for one or more hours while the iodine is absorbed. Your throat is then scanned with an instrument called a gamma camera, which detects the radioactivity from the iodine and produces an image of your thyroid gland. Thyroid scanning may be used to detect tumours or nodules in the thyroid, or after thyroid cancer surgery to detect any remaining cancer cells.

REPRODUCTIVE SYSTEM TESTS

Sperm count
A sperm count is considered normal if there are more than 15 million sperm per millilitre of semen, with over 50 per cent of the sperm able to swim effectively and over 30 per cent of normal shape.

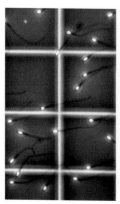
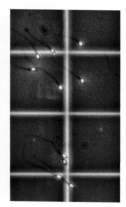

Normal sperm count   **Low sperm count**

Semen analysis
If a couple is struggling to conceive, their doctor may advise fertility tests. For the man, this involves a semen analysis to check the sperm. He provides a semen sample, which is sent to a laboratory where it is examined under a microscope to assess the number and health of the sperm. A low sperm count, or sperm that are abnormally shaped or not moving, can indicate a fertility problem. Men may also have semen analysis after a vasectomy, to check that they no longer have sperm in their semen.

Blood tests for sex hormones
Both men and women produce the sex hormones testosterone and oestrogen, but testosterone levels are naturally higher in men, and oestrogen levels are higher in women. Blood tests to assess levels of testosterone, oestrogen, and progesterone (a sex hormone produced only by women) may be used to investigate infertility; detect a sex hormone-producing tumour; or investigate erectile dysfunction in men, or menstrual problems or polycystic ovary syndrome in women. They may also be carried out to investigate early or delayed puberty in either sex, or premature menopause in women. In addition to checking levels of the sex hormones themselves, blood tests may also be carried out to check levels of luteinizing hormone (produced by the hypothalamus) and follicle-stimulating hormone (produced by the pituitary gland), because they help regulate production of the sex hormones.

Breast ultrasound scanning
If you find a lump in your breast, or if a lump is detected during a mammogram, an ultrasound scan of the breast may be carried out to investigate further. In this test, high-frequency sound waves are used to image the breast tissue. It can reveal the difference between fluid-filled cysts (which show as dark areas) and solid lumps (which appear pale). Ultrasound scanning may also used for guidance in tests such as a breast biopsy (see below). Ultrasound is quick, safe, and painless.

Breast biopsy
Biopsy involves taking a tissue sample for analysis. For a breast lump, you may have fine-needle aspiration, in which a thin needle is inserted into the lump to draw out a sample of cells or fluid. Other forms of biopsy include needle biopsy and punch biopsy, which involve taking larger samples; you may be given a local anaesthetic for these. The biopsy samples are then examined under a microscope to check for cancer. If you have a cyst, removing the fluid during the biopsy should make the cyst subside.

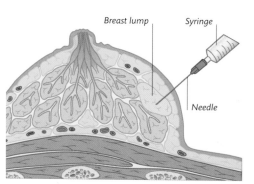

Breast lump   *Syringe*

Needle

Fine-needle aspiration of a breast lump
The lump is located by touch or ultrasound. A fine needle is inserted into it, and fluid or cells are drawn into the syringe.

SKIN AND SKELETAL SYSTEM TESTS

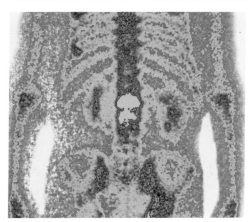

Bone density scan
This scan has been coloured to reveal areas of low (pink), medium (violet), and high (yellow) bone density. The large pink area in the spine indicates an area affected by osteoporosis.

Bone density scan
Also known as as DEXA scan, this procedure uses low-dose X-rays to assess the density of the bones. It is primarily used to diagnose osteoporosis, a condition that makes the bones weak and liable to break. Your doctor may advise a bone density scan if you are at risk of developing osteoporosis: for example, if you are a post-menopausal woman, if you smoke, if you have a kidney, liver, or thyroid disorder, or if you are taking medication that may cause bone loss, such as corticosteroids.

Skin biopsy
A skin biopsy involves taking a sample of abnormal skin to help diagnose diseases such as skin cancer, bacterial or fungal infections, or disorders such as psoriasis. A local anaesthetic is applied to the abnormal area and a sample is removed by scraping (shave biopsy) or cutting into deeper skin layers (excisional biopsy). In some cases, an entire lesion, such as a mole, may be removed. A small area of surrounding normal skin is usually also removed. The sample is then examined under a microscope for diagnosis.

NERVOUS SYSTEM TESTS

Brain imaging
Techniques such as computerized tomography (CT) scanning or magnetic resonance imaging (MRI) can be used to show the structures of the brain and reveal tumours or injured areas. Scans can also be used to show brain activity. For example, functional MRI (fMRI) can be used to show areas of increased activity when the brain performs various tasks. Positron emission tomography (PET scanning) may also be used to image brain activity. It involves injecting a radioactive tracer into a vein and then using a special scanner to detect the levels of radiation given off by different areas of the brain; the higher the radiation level, the more active the brain area.

EEG
Electroencephalography (EEG) is the measurement of electrical activity in the brain. It may be used to investigate seizures; sleep, memory, or behaviour problems; or brain damage. Electrodes are attached to your scalp to detect brain activity, which is displayed as a trace while you perform various tasks. Disorders show as abnormal EEG patterns.

Having an EEG
An EEG typically takes about 30 minutes and is painless. You will be asked to perform various simple tasks, such as opening and closing your eyes, while your brain activity is recorded.

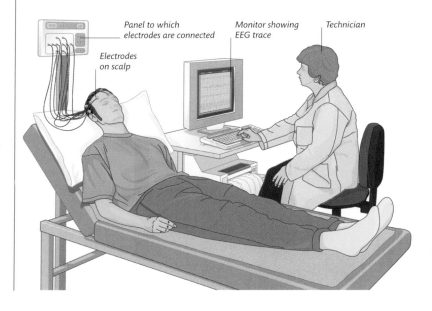

Panel to which electrodes are connected

Monitor showing EEG trace

Technician

Electrodes on scalp

Autonomic nervous system tests

The autonomic nervous system (ANS, see pp.132–33) controls many of the body's unconscious functions, such as the heartbeat and blood pressure. Problems affecting the ANS can cause various symptoms, such as fainting when you stand up, and may occur alone or as part of a disorder, such as Parkinson's disease. Tests to assess ANS function involve measuring your blood pressure, heart rate, and heart rhythm while you perform different exercises, including deep breathing, the Valsalva manoeuvre (blocking your nose and mouth and blowing out), and the tilt-table test (lying on a table as it is tilted).

Nerve conduction studies

These studies are used to investigate any disorder or injury that may disrupt nerve signals between your brain and limbs. They involve two tests, usually done together. In electromyography (EMG), a fine needle is inserted into a muscle to record the nerve signals while the muscle is resting and when it is active. Nerve conduction testing involves stimulating a nerve and then measuring the speed at which the nerve response signals travel along the nerve. The results of both tests are shown as traces on a monitor.

Nerve conduction testing
A technician stimulates a specific nerve and electrodes on your skin further along the path of that nerve detect the signals the nerve sends out. A computer analyses the signals and displays them as a trace.

Stimulator sends tiny electric impulse to nerve

Results displayed as a trace on monitor

Recording electrode

Technician

CHROMOSOME AND GENE TESTS

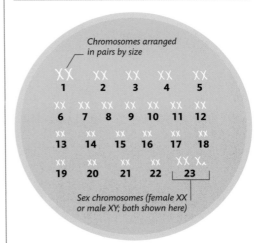

Chromosomes arranged in pairs by size

1 2 3 4 5
6 7 8 9 10 11 12
13 14 15 16 17 18
19 20 21 22 23

Sex chromosomes (female XX or male XY; both shown here)

Viewing the chromosomes
Chromosomes from a sample of blood or tissue are stained so that their shapes show up clearly. They are viewed under a microscope and sorted into 22 pairs of autosomes (non-sex chromosomes) and a single pair of sex chromosomes (XX for a female, or XY for a male) to produce an arrangement called a karyotype.

Chromosome tests

In normal body cells, the genetic material (DNA) is divided into 46 chromosomes, consisting of 22 pairs of autosomes (non-sex chromosomes) and one pair of sex chromosomes. In some disorders, however, a person is born with an extra, missing, or abnormal chromosome. Examples include Down's syndrome (also called trisomy 21), in which there is an extra copy of chromosome 21, and Turner's syndrome, in which a female has only one X chromosome instead of two, or one normal and one abnormal X chromosome. Chromosome testing is usually carried out only on people with signs of a chromosomal disorder, couples at risk of passing on a disorder, women who have repeated miscarriages, or unborn or newborn babies. A sample of blood (or amniotic fluid from a pregnant woman) is sent to a laboratory, where the chromosomes are separated and sorted by size to reveal any problems with their number or structure.

Gene tests

Some inherited conditions, such as cystic fibrosis and sickle cell disease, are caused by abnormalities in specific genes. You may be offered testing if your doctor suspects you have such a condition, if any close family members have a known or suspected genetic condition, or if you are at risk of passing on a genetic disorder to your children. Gene testing may also sometimes be offered to check for the presence for specific genes that are associated with an increased risk of developing certain conditions, such as the BRCA1 and BRCA2 genes associated with an increased risk of breast cancer. Commercial tests for many genetic conditions are also available. Testing usually requires only a blood sample or a scraping of cells from inside your cheek. For pregnant women, a sample of amniotic fluid or placental tissue may be used. The sample is sent to a laboratory, where it is processed to reveal any genetic abnormalities in the unborn baby. The results of gene tests may be difficult to interpret so it is advisable to discuss them with a genetic counsellor.

PSYCHOLOGICAL TESTS

Dependency assessment

Dependency is a problem with controlling your use of alcohol or drugs, or with behaviour such as compulsive sexual activity or gambling. It can be difficult for somebody to recognize dependency in themselves but there are various tests available to identify dependency and assess its severity. A doctor may ask questions about your lifestyle and may also use special questionnaires designed to give an insight into dependent behaviour. If alcohol or substance dependency is the problem, tests on your urine, blood, or hair may be carried out to determine the levels of alcohol or other substances in the body. Tests of organ function, such as liver-function tests (see p.71), may also be performed to check whether or not you have organ damage. The results of all these tests can be used as a basis for a personal care plan.

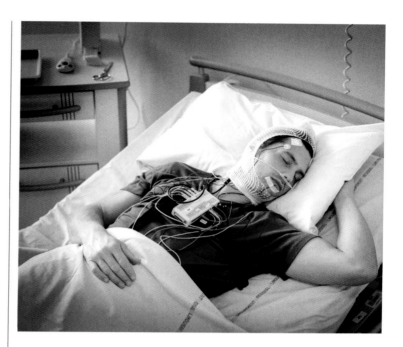

Sleep analysis

If you are suffering from a persistent inability to sleep, disturbed sleep patterns, or a problem such as snoring, your doctor may refer you to a sleep centre. There, specialists will assess you and may arrange tests to investigate specific aspects of your sleep. Some tests can be done at home, such as oximetry (wearing a monitor on your finger to measure blood oxygen levels while you sleep, see p.51), which may be used to detect problems such as obstructive sleep apnoea. In this condition, the walls of the throat relax and become narrowed during sleep, which interrupts breathing and may also cause snoring. For other tests, such as polysomnography, you will have to stay in the sleep centre overnight. Polysomnography shows when you fall asleep and which stages of sleep you pass through. It also measures several basic body functions, such as your breathing, and your brain activity. You may be monitored with a video camera, to show your sleep position and any unusual activity patterns. Further tests may be carried out the day after your sleep, to assess your level of wakefulness.

Polysomnography
In this test, you sleep at a sleep centre. You are connected to various monitors to measure your brain waves, eye movements, muscle activity, heart rate, and breathing.

Health screening options

It can be challenging to decide which health checks to have and when to have them. The information here gives examples of recommendations for adults in various countries, which may help to make you aware of possible options to consider.

Choosing tests

Many countries have health screening programmes, the recommendations of which vary depending on the health needs of their particular populations. Most screening programmes for adults are to do with cancer prevention.

Some countries also have legally required health checks for certain groups (see pp.16–19). For example, in Japan there are mandatory annual health check-ups for full-time employees, an annual stress test for employees, and an annual health check-up for people aged between 40 and 74 that specifically aims to prevent lifestyle-related diseases. In addition, there may be legally required checks in certain countries for specific jobs, such as drivers, or for workers who may be exposed to potentially hazardous substances. Some employers may also require employees to undergo health checks as a condition of employment.

The information below gives examples of recommendations for key optional health checks for adults in selected countries. Not included are screening tests for specific groups with special health needs, such as pregnant women or people with diabetes. It is important to note that individual health needs differ, and the information here is not intended as a substitute for expert medical advice.

It is also important to be informed about what is available and appropriate for you and you should always consult a healthcare professional about your own personal health matters.

BLOOD AND CIRCULATORY SYSTEM

• **Blood pressure**. In the UK, a blood pressure test at least every five years is advised for all those over 40 years old. The US recommends checks for all adults, but especially older adults, every one to two years. In Australia, all men over 18 years old are advised to have their blood pressure tested at least once every two years. In Canada, blood pressure is usually checked as an adult during a routine doctor visit. The frequency of checks depends on age and other health factors, but checks are generally advised at least once every two to three years.

• **Blood glucose**. Recommendations vary considerably about the frequency of testing in the UK and Australia. In the US, testing is recommended from 45 years old for those at risk of pre-diabetes or of developing diabetes in the future. In Canada, testing is generally advised from the age of 40.

• **Blood cholesterol**. In the UK, blood cholesterol checks are generally recommended for those who suffer from high blood pressure or diabetes; they may also be advised for people with a family history of high blood pressure or high cholesterol, or those who are 40 years old and/or overweight and have never had their cholesterol levels checked before. In the US, testing once every five years is advised for younger adults, and every one to two years for men aged 45–65 and women aged 55–65. Australia recommends testing every five years for people aged 45 and above. In Canada, testing is generally advised every two years for adults over 40, although the recommended frequency depends on individual health factors.

• **Abdominal aortic aneurysm**. In the UK, an ultrasound scan for abdominal aortic aneurysm is offered to men at the age of 65. There is no formal screening for the condition in most other countries. However, in the US, Canada, and Australia, a scan is available on request for those who may be at risk – from 60 years old in Australia, and from 65 years old in the US and Canada.

DIGESTIVE SYSTEM AND ORAL HEALTH

• **Bowel cancer screening**. Older adults are generally recommended to be screened for bowel cancer, typically either with a faecal test or bowel endoscopy (direct examination of the bowel with a flexible viewing tube). Some countries have national screening programmes for bowel cancer, specific details of which vary between countries. For example, in the UK, many men and women are offered one-off bowel endoscopy at the age of 55, then a faecal test every two years from the ages of 60 to 74. In Italy, a faecal test is offered every two years to those aged 50–69, although in Piedmont, a one-off bowel endoscopy is offered to those aged 58–60. In France, a faecal test is offered every two years to those aged 50–74. In Australia, screening is also offered every two years, but for men and women between the ages of 50 and 64. In the US, annual screening is advised for men and women between the ages of 50 and 75. In Canada, men and women over the age of 50 are advised to have a faecal test every two years or bowel endoscopy every 10 years.

- **Dental check-up**. In the UK and US, it is recommended to have regular dental check-ups anywhere from once every three months to once every two years, depending on the health of the individual's teeth and gums. In Canada, the general recommendation is to have a dental check-up once or twice a year.

MUSCULOSKELETAL SYSTEM AND SKIN

- **Bone density scan**. In the US, women are advised to have annual bone density scans to check for osteoporosis from the age of 65, and men from the age of 70. In Canada, bone density scans are recommended for men and women over 65. In Australia and the UK, bone density scans are only recommended for people who are at increased risk of developing osteoporosis, for those over 35 in Australia, or those over 50 in the UK.
- **Skin cancer check**. In the UK, the National Health Service advises visiting your doctor if you notice a change in the appearance of your moles (for example, in their size, shape, or colour) or if you develop any new moles. These changes may indicate melanoma, a type of malignant skin cancer. The advice is the same in Australia and Canada.

REPRODUCTIVE SYSTEM

- **Cervical screening**. In the UK, the National Health Service invites women for their first cervical screening up to six months before their 25th birthday, then every three years from 25–49, and finally once every five years for those aged 50–64. In France, and Italy, women aged 25–64 are offered cervical screening using a smear every three years, although those aged 30–64 may be offered screening using the test for HPV (human papillomavirus) once every five years instead. In the US, all women are advised to begin cervical screening at age 21, with screening once every three years until 30 years old, and then once every five years until the age of 65. In Australia, women aged 25–74 are invited for a cervical screening test two years after their last cervical smear test, and then once every five years. In Canada, women aged 25–69 are advised to have a cervical screening test once every three years.
- **Breast cancer screening**. In the UK, all women aged 50–71 and registered with their GP are invited for a breast cancer szcreening every three years. In France and Australia, women aged 50–74 are offered screening every two years. In Italy, screening is generally offered every two years to women aged 50–69, although in some regions screening is offered once a year for women aged 45–49, then every two years from 50–74. In the US, the American Cancer Society recommends annual breast cancer screening for women aged 45–54, then once every two years for women aged 55 and older. In Canada, women aged 50–75 are offered breast cancer screening once every two years.

- **Sexually transmitted infections**. In the UK, it is advised that people who think they may be at risk of an STI (for example, because they have had unprotected sex with a new partner) should be tested for STIs, even if they do not have symptoms. In the US, the Centers for Disease Control and Prevention recommends that all individuals aged 13–64 should be tested at least once in their lifetime for HIV, and once a year for anyone who practises unsafe sex. In Canada, annual screening for chlamydia and gonorrhoea is recommended for sexually active people under 25; for those older than 25 and who are at risk of infection, screening every three years is advised. Screening for HIV is also recommended for all those at risk of infection.

EYES AND VISION

- **Eye tests**. In the UK, US, and Australia, it is generally advised to have an eye test every two years. However, in the US, additional screenings are also advised. These include a baseline eye disease screening at age 40 for those not showing symptoms and not in an at-risk category (for example, due to a family history of eye disease such as glaucoma). In the US, the National Institutes of Health also recommends an annual dilated eye examination from the age of 60 onwards. In Canada, eye tests are recommended every five years between the ages of 20 and 39, every two years between the ages of 40 and 64, then annually for those aged 65 or older.

Vaccination record

It is useful to keep a record of vaccinations, noting information such as that in the example below. You can copy the charts to record information about every member of the family.

NAME:

Date	Vaccine	Stage/dose of vaccine	Next dose(s) due
12 June 2019	Typhoid (oral)	1st dose of 3	2nd dose due 14 June 2019; 3rd dose due 16 June 2019

Date	Vaccine	Stage/dose of vaccine	Next dose(s) due

Weight record

Many people find it useful to keep a record of their weight, to ensure they remain a healthy weight or to monitor weight changes. You can copy the blank chart and use a copy for each person. If you want to calculate your body mass index, see pp.24–25.

NAME:

Date and time	Weight	Body mass index (BMI)	Notes
12 June 2019, 9a.m.	75kg/165lb	24.0	At top end of healthy range

Blood pressure record

This chart enables you to record blood pressure (see pp.28–31), however frequently you need to measure it. If you are taking it at home, do it at the same time of day every time as blood pressure fluctuates throughout the day.

NAME:

Date and time	Systolic pressure	Diastolic pressure	Notes
12 June 2019, 9a.m.	120mm Hg	80mm Hg	Within normal range; check again in evening

Health checks record

This chart enables you to record the medical checks you and other members of your family have had. You can copy the blank charts and use a copy for each member of the family.

NAME:

Date	Test	Result	Notes
12 June 2019	Mammography	Normal	Next mammogram due in 3 years

Date	Test	Result	Notes

Index

Page numbers in **bold** refer to main entries.

A

abdominal aortic aneurism scan **40–41**, 176
abdominal muscles 126, 129
abdominal ultrasound **70**
abscesses 99
acne 99
ACR (albumin:creatinine ratio) 75, 76
addictive substances **150–51**
ADH (antidiuretic hormone) 73
adrenal glands 72, 73, 133
adrenaline 63
aerobic exercise 164
ageing
  age-related mental changes 141
  and exercise 154–55
  and health 13
agility 153, 156
AIDS 53
air
  breathing 42, 43, 45
  clean 12
AKI (acute kidney injury) 77
albumin 71, 75, 76
alcohol **150**
  and blood pressure 31
  and bones 156
  and cholesterol 59
  dependency assessment **175**
  and fertility 163
  and health 14
  and heart 34
  and kidneys 77
  and psychological health 164
  and skin 158
  and teeth 119
aldosterone 73
alimentary canal 64, 65
allergens 62, 63

allergic rhinitis 62
allergies 17, 53, **62–63**, 170
alveoli 42, 43
ambulatory ECG 34
amino acids 146
amygdala 139
amylase 64
anaemia 55, 71
anaphylactic shock 63
aneurysms 170
  aortic 27, **40–41**, 177
angina 154
angiography **170**
ankle rotation 125
ante-natal care 87
antibodies 52, 53, 61, 80, 144, 170
antigens 80
anus 88
anxiety 31, 32, 140, 141, 164, 165
aorta 26, 40
aortic aneurysm 27, **40–41**, 177
applanation tonometry 109
armpits 94
arteries 26, 27
  angiography 170
  blood pressure 28
  carotid artery Doppler scan **169**
  cholesterol 58, 59
  narrowing 31, 37
arthritis 122, 155
asthma 20, 45, 47, 49, 62
astigmatism 102, **104**
asymptomatic conditions 10
athlete's foot 99, 158
atrial fibrillation 34
at-risk groups, tests for **19**
atrium 26
audiogram 112
audiometry **112**
auditory cortex 138
auditory nerve 110, 111
autoimmune disorders 53, 55
autonomic nervous system **132–33**, 134
  tests **174**
autosomes 174
axons 130, 131

B

Babinski foot reflex test 134
"back-scratch" test 124
bacteria
  bacterial skin infections 158, 173
  Helicobacter pylori **68–69**
  STIs 80–81
  teeth 117
  in urine 74, 75
balance **134**, 137, 153, 156
  ears and 110, **111**
ball-and socket joints 121
basal ganglia 132
B cells 52, 53
bedtime routine 165
behavioural factors **14–15**
Beighton Score 124
benchpress exercises 129
biceps 122
bicycles, exercise 51
bile 58, 65
bile ducts 71
bilirubin 75
biopsies
  breast 95, 172
  cervix 91
  lung 170
  prostate 83
  skin 173
  testicles 83
bird-dog exercise 126
biting 117
bladder 72, 83
blinking 100
blisters 99
blood **52–53**
  blood clotting factors 61, 71
  blood count **55**
  blood flow 39, 169
  blood glucose levels 21, **56–57**, 128, 137, 176
  blood samples 54, 56, 59
  and breathing **42–43**
  cholesterol tests **58–59**, 176
  circulatory system **26–27**
  digestive system 65
  exercise capacity **50–51**
  filtering by kidneys 72–73

blood *continued*
  oxygenation **51**
  in stools 66
  in urine 74, 75
blood pressure 27, 153, 176
  and aortic aneurysm 40, 41
  echocardiography 39
  and heart 34
  and kidneys 77
  measuring 21, **28–31**, 32, 36
  records 181
blood tests 53, **60–61**, 176
  for allergies **170**
  blood cholesterol **58–59**
  blood count **55**
  blood glucose **56–57**
  gynaecological infections 88, 89
  hormonal disorders 85
  kidney function 73, 77
  liver function **71**
  for mood analysis 141
  for sex hormones **172**
  STIs **80–81**, 85, 88, 89
blood vessels 26, 31, 37, 40, 52, 133
BMI (body mass index) 24, **25**, 156, 163
body temperature 96
boils 99
bones
  bone density scans 122, **173**, **177**
  decreasing bone mass 156
  healthy **156–57**
  keeping fit 152, 153, 154
  skeleton **120–21**
  X-rays 44
bowel
  cancer screening **66–67**, **176–77**
  scope screening 67
brain
  and alcohol 150
  and balance 111
  dementia testing **140–41**
  EEG **173**
  and hearing 110
  how the mind works **138–39**

brain *continued*
  imaging **173**
  nervous system **130–33**
  and vision 100
breasts 84, 85
  biopsy **172**
  breast cancer 61, 85, **94–95**,
    172, 175, 177
  mammograms 85, 94, **95**
  ultrasound scanning **172**
breathing **42–43**, **45**, **46–47**
  exercises 165
  pattern 48
breathlessness 34, 37, 39, 50
breath sample 69
Broca's area 138
bronchoscopy **170**
bruises 99

C

caffeine 32
calcium 61, 122, 146, 156, 157
calluses 99
calories
  in alcohol 150
  in food 58, 148–49
cancer
  and alcohol 150
  blood count 55
  blood tests 61
  bowel **66–67**, **176–77**
  breast 85, **94–95**, 172, 177
  cancer cells 53
  cervical 85, **92–93**, 177
  and exercise 155
  prostate 61, 79, **83**
  skin 97, 98, 159, 173, 177
  and smoking 151
  testicular 79, **82**
  tumour marker
    tests **170–71**
  urine analysis 75
capillaries 26, 27, 43, 72, 96
carbohydrates 146, 149
carbon dioxide 42, 43, 69
carbon isotopes 69
cardiopulmonary exercise (CPEX)
  testing **50–51**

cardiovascular disease 27
  and alcohol 150
  cardiovascular system tests
    169–70
  and drug use 151
  and exercise 154, 155
  high blood pressure 30, 31
  and weight 24
carotid artery Doppler
  scan **169**
cartilage 44, 120
cataracts 106
cavities, dental 117, 118
cells
  blood glucose levels 56–57
  cell membranes 58
  pre-cancerous 92, 93
central nervous system (CNS)
  130, 132
cerebellum 132, 139
cerebral cortex 132
cervical vertebrae 120
cervix 90
  cervical cancer 85, **92–93**
  cervical screening test 90, 91,
    92–93, **177**
  colposcopy **91**, 93
chambers, heart 26
chaperones 90, 93
chest
  CT scan **169**
  MRI scan **169**
  pain 34, 37, 39
  X-rays 43, **44**
chewing 117
chickenpox 145
chlamydia 80, 81, 163, 177
cholera 144
cholesterol
  blood tests 53, **58–59**, 176
  high 40
  types of 148
choroid 101
chromosome tests **174**
chronic obstructive pulmonary
  disease *see* COPD
chyme 64
circulatory system **26–27**, 152,
  176
CKD (chronic kidney disease) 77

closed-chain exercises 129
clotting 52, 53
coccyx 120
cochlea 111
coeliac disease 61
cognitive function 112,
  140–41
cold sores 99
collagen 122
collarbones 121
colon 64
colonoscopy 66, 67
colour vision test **105**
colposcopy **91**, 93
commercial testing **21**
common aneurysm 40
complete blood
  count (CBC) 55
compulsive behaviours 175
conception 86
condoms 162–63
cone cells 100, 101
connective tissues 120, 122
conscious thought 138
contact dermatitis 63
contact lenses 104
contraception 162, 163
contraction, muscles 122
coordination 133, **134–35**, 156
COPD (chronic obstructive
  pulmonary disease) 47, 49, 55
core muscles 123
core stability testing **126–27**
cornea 100, 102, 104, 109
corns 99
corpora cavernosa 78, 79
corpus spongiosum 78, 79
cortex 132, 138, 139
cortisol 165
CPEX *see* cardiopulmonary
  exercise testing
cranial nerves 130
creatinine 75, 76, 77
CT (computed tomography)
  scans 169, 173
curl-ups 129
cystic fibrosis 175
cysts
  breast 172
  ovarian 90

cysts *continued*
  skin 99
  testicular 82
cytokines 62
cytology 93

D

deafness 110
decibels 112, 113
declarative memory 139
dehydration 73, 77, 146
dementia 112, 139, 152
  testing for **140–41**
dendrites 131
dental checks 117,
  118–19, 177
dentine 117
dependency assessment **175**
depression 112, 139, 140, 141,
  150, 152, 165
depth perception 100
dermis 96
dermoscopy 98
DEXA scans **173**
diabetes 24, 101, 148, 149, 155,
  158, 176
  blood glucose levels 20, 54,
    56–57
  and eye health 106
  pre-diabetes 10
  type 2 148, 149, 152
  urine analysis 74, 75, 76
  and weight 24
diagnostic tests **18**
diaphragm 42, 43, 126
diastolic blood pressure 28, 29,
  30, 31
diet
  adapting **148–49**
  allergy testing **170**
  and aortic aneurysm 41
  and blood pressure 31
  and fertility 163
  and health 14
  healthy **146–47**
  and heart 32, 34
  and keeping fit 152
  and mood 140

diet *continued*
and psychological
health 164
safeguarding bones and
muscles 156, 157
and skin 99, 158
and teeth 119
and vision 103, 161
and weight 25
digestive system 58,
64-65, 132
bowel cancer screening **66-67**
H. pylori testing **68-69**
mouth and teeth **116-17**
MRI scan **171**
tests **171**, **176-77**
digital rectal examination 83
diphtheria 145
dipstick tests 75, 76
discs, intervertebral 120
dissecting aneurysm 40
dizziness 30, 34
DNA (deoxyribonucleic acid) 79
Doppler scans 39
Down's syndrome 174
driving, and vision 108
drugs 150, **151**
dependency assessment **175**
and health 14
and psychological
health 164
duodenum 64, 65, 171
dynamic resistance 128

E

early detection 10, 94, 95
ears 138
cleaning 160
ear canal 110, 115, 160
ear defenders 160
eardrum 110, 111,
114-15, 160
ear tests **110**
earwax 110, 114, 160
health **160**
hearing tests **112-13**
tympanometry **114-15**
working of **110-11**

ECG 27, **34-35**, 51
exercise **36-37**
echocardiography 27, **38-39**
eczema 62, 63, 99, 158
EEG (electroencephalography)
173
eGFR (estimated glomerular
filtration rate) 77
eggs 78, 84, 85, 86
elbows 122
electrocardiogram *see* ECG
electrolytes 77
electronic cigarettes 151
ellipsoidal joints 121
Ely test 124
EMG (electromyography) 125,
174
emotions 138, 139
promoting positive 164
enamel, tooth **117**
endocrine system 73
tests **171**
endometrium 84, 85
endoscopy 176-77
endurance 153
energy density,
food 148-49
environmental factors **12**
enzymes 61, 64, 65, 71, 116
epidermis 96, 97
epididymis 79, 82
epiglottis 116
episodic memory 139
equipment, home
monitoring **21**
erectile dysfunction 172
essential fatty acids 146, 147
ethnicity 13
Eustachian tube 111, 114, 115
exclusion diets **170**
exercise
and aortic aneurysm 41
and blood pressure 31
and cholesterol 59
for core stability 126
exercise capacity 43, **50-51**
exercise ECG 34, **36-37**
and fertility 163
and health 14
and heart health 34

exercise *continued*
and heart rate 32
keeping fit **152-53**
and mood 140
muscle strength and endurance
128-29
and psychological health 164,
165
safeguarding bones and
muscles **156-57**
for special groups **154-55**
and weight 25
exhalation 42, 43, 47
extensor muscles 122
eyes 132, 138, 139
astigmatism **104**
colour vision test **105**
eyebrows 100
eye health 101, **106-7**, **161**
eyelashes 100
eyelids 100
eye pressure **109**
and high blood pressure 31
testing vision **102-3**, **177**
visual field **108**
working of **100-101**

F

faeces 64
faecal antigen test 68
faecal immunochemical test
(FIT) 66
faecal microscopy **171**
faecal occult blood test (FOB)
66
fallopian tubes 84
falls 153, 156
false-positive/negative results
10, 11
family medical history 13
Farnsworth D-15 test 105
fascicles 130
fasting blood tests 54, 57, 59
fat
cholesterol 58, 59
dietary 146, 147
digestive system 65
distribution 24, 25

fat *continued*
excess 24
reducing saturated 149
feet
foot care **158**
testing sensory nerve pathways
136-37
female reproductive system
84-85
colposcopy **91**
infections **88-89**
pelvic examination **90**
pregnancy testing **86-87**
ferritin 61
fertility
maximizing **163**
tests 172
fertilization 78, 84,
85, 86
fetus 85
fibre 146
fibrin 53
field of vision 102
fight or flight 132
finger-pricking technique 54, 57,
58
finger-to-nose test 134, 135
fitness **152-53**
FITTR 152, 155
flexibility **124**, 126, 153
flexor muscles 122
fluid balance 73
focal length 100
folic acid 87
follicles
hair 96
ovaries 84
follicle-stimulating hormone
(FSH) 85
folliculitis 99
food
allergies 63
digestive system 64-65
healthy diet **146-47**
H. pylori 69
mouth and teeth 116, 117
foot care **158**
forearm planks 126
fractures 122, 156
frequencies 112, 113

fruit and vegetables 146, 147
full blood count (FBC) 55, 71
fungal infections 97, 99,
    158, 173

G

gait 124, **125**
gallbladder 65, 70, 71
gallstones 70, 71
gas exchange 42, 43
gastroscopy **171**
gender 13
gene tests **175**
genetics 13, 19
genital herpes 80, 163
genital warts 80
glass test 99
glaucoma 101, 108, 109
gliding joints 121
glomerulus 72, 73
glucose 53
    blood glucose levels 54, **56–57**
    urine tests 75
gluteal muscles 126
glycosylated haemoglobin 56
goals, personal 164
goggles 161
gonorrhoea 80, 163, 177
GP health checks **16**
gravity 110, 111
grip strength 122, 128
gums 117, 118, 119, 146
gynaecological infections **88–89**

H

haematocrit 55
haemoglobin 51, 52, 55, 56
hair cells, ears 111
hair follicles 96
hamstrings 124
hands 136, 137
hard palate 116
hayfever 62
HbA1c test 56
HDLs (high-density lipoproteins)
    58, 59, 148

health checks
    DIY **20–21**
    records 182–83
    types of **16–17**
hearing 110–15
    age-related hearing loss 110,
        160
    hearing aids 113
    protecting **160**
    tests **112–13**
heart
    blood pressure **28–31**
    breathing **42–43**
    cardiovascular system tests
        169–70
    checking heart rate **32–33**
    cholesterol tests **58–59**
    circulatory system **26–27**
    ECG **34–35**
    echocardiography **38–39**
    exercise capacity **50–51**
    exercise ECG **36–37**
    heart attacks 27, 31, 32, 34, 37,
        39
    heart disease see cardiovascular
        disease
    heart failure 39
    heart murmurs 39
    keeping fit 152, **153**
    nervous system 133
    size 44
heartbeat 28
    rhythm of **34–35**
heart rate 27
    checking **32–33**
    CPEX 50–51
    and exercise 155
    exercise ECG 37
height 13, 25
Helicobacter pylori **68–69**
hepatitis A 144
hepatitis B 80, 81, 88, 144
hepatitis C 80
hernias 70
high blood pressure 28, 30–31,
    39, 40
hinge joints 121
hip girdle muscles 126
hippocampus 139
hip size 24

histamine 62
HIV 55, 80, 81, 88, 163, 177
hormones 52, 56, 57, 58, 61, 146
    blood tests for sex hormones
        172
    female reproductive system
        84, 85
    kidneys 73
    male reproductive system 79
    pregnancy 87
housing, quality of 12
HPV 92, 93, 145, 158, 163, 177
human chorionic gonadotropin
    (hCG) 87
human papillomavirus see HPV
hydration 146, 158
hygiene
    eyes 161
    H. pylori 69
    skin 158
hyperlordosis 125
hypermetropia 102
hypermobility 124
hypertension 28, 30–31, 39, 75
hypodermis 96

I

ileum 64
immune system **53**
    and allergies **62–63**, **170**
    tests **170–71**
    vaccinations **144–45**
immunodeficiency 53
immunoglobulins 52, 144, 170
impact, exercise 157
implicit memory 139
income, and health 15
incus (anvil) bone 111
indigestion 68
infections
    checking for **80–81**
    and drug use 151
    role of blood 52, 53, 61
    skin 158
    vaccinations **144–45**
infertility 163
inflammation 61
influenza 144, 145

inhalation 42, 43
inherited conditions 175
injury prevention 134, 136
inner ear 110, 111, 114
insect bites 99, 158
insulin 56, 57, 65
insurance companies, health
    checks 17
intolerances 17
iris 100, 109
Ishihara test 105

J

Japanese encephalitis 144
jaws 116, 117, 118
jejenum 64
joints **120–21**, 152, 154
    flexibility, posture, and gait
        124–25

K

karyotypes 174
keratometer 104
ketones 75, 76
kidneys **72–73**
    abdominal ultrasound 70
    chemicals produced by 53
    function tests 61, 73, **76–77**
    and high blood pressure 31
    urine analysis 74, 75
knee reflex 135
kyphoscoliosis 47
kyphosis 125

L

lactic acid 117
language 138, 139
large intestine 64
lateral bridge 127
lazy eye 101
LDLs (low-density lipoproteins)
    58, 59, 148
learning 138, **139**
legpress exercise 128, 129

leisure 15
lens 100, 102
leukaemia 55
lifestyle 15
lifting 156
ligaments 120, 124, 126
light receptor cells 100, 101
light-touch test 136
limbic association area 138
lipoproteins 58, 59
liver 65, 152, 171
    abdominal ultrasound 70
    chemicals produced by 53
    cholesterol 58, 59
    function tests 60, 61, **71**
    liver failure 150
long-sightedness 102, 104
long-term conditions 18
low blood pressure 30
low mood 140, 141
lumbar vertebrae 120
lunges 129
lungs 28, 133
    breathing **42–43**
    chest X-ray **44**
    exercise capacity **50–51**
    function tests 43
    keeping fit 152, 153
    lung volume tests 43, **48–49**
    normal immune response 62
    peak flow **45**
    respiratory system tests **169–70**
    role of blood 52
    spirometry **46–47**
    whole-body plethysmography **48–49**
luteinizing hormone (LH) 85
lymphocytes 52, 53

M

macular degeneration 106
male reproductive system **78–79**
    checking the prostate **83**
    checking the testicles **82**
    infections **80–81**
malleus (hammer) bone 111

mammograms 85, 94, **95**
masseter muscle 122
mast cells 62
measles 145
medical checks **18–19**, 176
medical history 13, 17
medicals, preparing for **17**
medications, regular 17
melanin 96, 97
melanocytes 97
melanoma 98
melatonin 165
memory 138, **139**
meningitis 99, 144, 145
menopause 85, 156, 172
menstrual cycle 84, 85, 87
mental health **138–41**, 152
    dementia testing **140–41**
    mood analysis **140–41**
    psychological health **164–65**
metabolism 24
microalbumin 75, 76
microvilli 65
middle ear 110, 114–15
milk 84, 85
mind-body connection 164
mind, working of **138–39**
minerals 61, 146, 147
miscarriages 174
mobile phones, health apps 34
moisturizer 158
moles 20, 98, 173
monitoring, advantages and disadvantages **10–11**
mood analysis **140–41**
motor cortex 138
motor nerves 132, 133
mouth 42, 64, **116–17**, 132, 138
movement
    and brain 138, 139
    and muscles 122
    and skeleton 121
MRA (magnetic resonance angiography) **169**
MRI (magnetic resonance imaging) scans 83, 168, 169, 171, 173
multifidus 126

mumps 145
muscles **122–23**
    brain and 138
    core stability testing **126–27**
    flexibility, posture and gait **124–25**
    healthy **156–57**
    keeping fit 152, 153
    loss of mass 122
    strength and endurance **128–29**
    wasting 77
musculoskeletal checks **122**, **126–27**, **177**
myelin sheaths 130, 131

N

neck pulse 32, 33
nephrons 72, 73
nerves 130–33, 138
    nerve cells *see* neurons
    nerve conduction studies **174**
nervous system **130–33**
    testing 133, **173–74**
    testing reflexes **134–35**
    testing sensory nerve pathways **136–37**
neurons 101, 111, 131
neurotransmitters 131
neutrophils 53
nicotine replacement therapy 151
nipples 85, 94
nitrates 75
non-medical interventions 10
nose 42
nuclear scans 37
numbness 136
nutrients 26, 64, 65, 146–49

O

obesity 47, 155
obstructive lung disease 47, 49
obstructive sleep apnoea 175
occipital lobe 139
occupation, and health 15

ocular hypertension 109
oesophagus 64, 116, 171
oestrogen 85, 87, 172
online testing **21**
open-chain exercises 129
ophthalmoscope 107
optic nerve 100, 101, 109
optometrists 102–9
oral health **117**, 119, **177**
ossicles 110, 111, 114
osteoporosis 24, 154, 155, 157, 173, 177
ovaries 84, 85, 90
    ovarian cancer 61
    ovarian cysts 61
    ovulation 84, 85, 87
oximetry 43, **51**, 175
oxygen 26, 42, 43, 52
    saturation 51

P

pain-type test 136
palpitations 34, 37
pancreas 56, 57, 65, 171
panic attacks 140
paraspinal muscles 126
parasympathetic system 132–33
parietal lobe 139
Parkinson's disease 174
parotid gland 116
patch testing **63**
pathogens 53
peak flow tests 21, 43, **44**
pelvis 120, 121, 124, 126
    pelvic examination **90**, 93
    pelvic floor muscles 126
    pelvic inflammation 163
penis 78, 79
perimetry 108
periods *see* menstrual cycle
peripheral nervous system (PNS) 130
peripheral neuropathy 136, 137
peripheral vision 108, 109
peristalsis 64, 65
personal factors **13**

personal fitness monitors **21**, 32, 51, 152, 154
personal heart rate monitors 32
personality 138
pertussis (whooping cough) 145
PET scans (positron emission tomography) 173
phagocytes 52, 53
phoropter 103, 104
phosphate 61
pH, urine 75
physical activity
    see exercise
physiotherapy 125
pinna 110
pin-prick test 136
pituitary gland 73, 85
pivot joints 121
plaque
    arterial 58, 59
    dental 117, 118
plasma 52, 53
platelets 52, 53, 55
plethysmography, whole-body **48–49**
pleural membrane 42
pneumonia 150
polio 145
pollution 12
polycystic ovary syndrome 172
polyps 67
polysomnography 175
portion size 148
position sense 137
postural stability 153
posture 124, **125**
pre-conditions 10
pre-existing conditions, monitoring **18**
prefrontal cortex 138, 139
pregnancy 85
    contraception 162, 163
    testing for **86–87**
    and X-rays 44
premotor cortex 138
presbyopia 102, 103, 104
primary visual cortex 139
progesterone 84, 85, 87, 172
pronation 125
proprioception 137

prostate gland 78, 83
    checking **83**
    prostate cancer 61, 79, **83**
    tests 83
proteins
    in blood 61, 71
    and bone and muscle health 156, 157
    dietary 146, 147
    in urine 75, 76
PSA (prostate-specific-antigen) tests 83
psoriasis 99, 173
psychological health **164–65**
    psychological tests **175**
puberty 85
public transport 12
pulmonary fibrosis 49
pulse **32–33**
    irregular 31, 32
    pulse oximetry 43, **51**
pupils 100, 109
    dilation of 107
push-ups 129
putamen 139

Q
quadriceps 124
questionnaires 139

R
rabies 144
rectum 67
    digital rectal examination 83
red blood cells 51, 52, 55, 75
reflexes 133
    testing **134–35**
refraction testing 102, 106
rehabilitation programmes 124, 126, 127, 155
relationships 15, 164
renal vein 72
reproductive system
    female **84–95**
    male **78–83**
    tests **172, 177**

resistance training **129**, 153, 154
restrictive lung disease 47, 49
retina 100, 101
    retinal photography 107
ribcage 120
ringworm 99
RNA (ribonucleic acid) 80
rod cells 101
rubella 145

S
sacrum 120, 126
saddle joints 121
safer sex 81, 88, **162–63**
saliva 64, 80, 116
salt, reducing dietary 77, 149
salts, and kidneys 73, 77
sclera 101
scoliosis 125
screening **18**
    options **176–77**
sebaceous glands 96
seborrhoeic dermatitis 99
sebum 97
self-help measures
    alcohol, tobacco and drugs **150–51**
    aortic aneurysm 41
    blood pressure 31
    bones and muscles **156–57**
    cholesterol levels 59
    dental health 119
    diet **146–49**
    ear health **160**
    exercise **152–55**
    eye health 103, **161**
    heart rate 32
    kidney function 77
    lung function 47
    psychological health 140, **164–65**
    sexual health 81, 88, **162–63**
    skin health 99, **158–59**
    vaccinations **144–45**
    weight 25

self monitoring
    blood cholesterol 58
    blood glucose 57
    blood oxygenation 51
    blood pressure 31
    breast awareness 94
    DIY health checks **20–21**
    ECG 34
    equipment **21**
    heart health 31, 32, 34, 58
    personal fitness monitors **21**, 32, 51, 152, 154
    pregnancy 87
    STIs 81
    teeth and mouth 119
    testicles 82
semen 78, 83
    analysis **172**
seminiferous tubules 79
sensory association cortex 139
sensory nerves 132, 133, 134
    testing pathways **136–37**
sex chromosomes 174
sex hormones 172
sexual health 15, **162–63**
sexual intercourse 78, 84
sexually transmitted infections (STIs) 79, **80–81**, **88–89**, 162–63, **177**
shingles 145
short-sightedness 102, 104
shoulder blades 121
sickle cell disease 175
sight *see* vision
sigmoidoscopy 67
single-leg squat 127
sit-and-reach test 124
skeleton **120–21**
    and muscles 122–23
    posture **125**
    skeletal system tests **173**
skin **96–97**, 133, 138
    biopsy **173**
    checking 97, **98–99**

skin *continued*
  colour 97
  healthy **158–59**
  infections spread by skin-to-
    skin contact 163
  skin cancer 97,
    98, 159, 173, 177
  and tobacco 151
skin prick testing **63**
skull 120, 121
sleep 152
  analysis **175**
  and health 14
  and mood 140
  and psychological health 164,
    165
  and skin 158
  and weight 25
slit lamps 106–7
small intestine 64, 65
smart phones 51
smart watches 32, 34
smear tests 85,
    92–93, **177**
smoking **151**
  and aortic aneurysm 40, 41
  and bone health 156
  and breathing 47
  and cholesterol 59
  and fertility 163
  and health 14
  and heart 32, 34
  and kidneys 77
  and psychological health
    164
  and skin 99, 158
  and teeth 119
  and vision 103, 161
Snellen chart 102
social connections 164
social life 15
soft palate 116
somatosensory cortex 138
sound waves 39, 110, 111, 114,
    115
spatial memory 139
specific gravity, urine 75
speech 138
  speech perception
    test **113**

sperm 78, 79, 84, 86, 172
sphygmomanometer 29
spinal cord 130, 131, 133, 134,
    137
spine **120**,
    121, 126
  curvature 125
spirometry 43, 45, **46–47**,
    48, 49, 51
spleen 70
sport, health checks 17
squints 101
stapes (stirrup)
    bone 111
static resistance 128
STIs *see* exually transmitted
    infections
stomach 64, 65,
    171
  ulcers 65, 68
stress 15, 31,
    32, 152
  exercise ECG
    (stress test) 37
  and mood 140
  and psychological health 164,
    165
  and skin 158
  of tests 11
  and weight 25
strokes 27
  cholesterol 56
  high blood pressure
    30
sublingual gland 116
submandibular
    gland 116
sugars, dietary 149
sunburn 99
sunglasses 161
sunlight 97, 157, 158, 159
sunscreen 159
superficial muscles 123
supination 125
support networks 165
swabs
  cervical 90
  urethral 81
  vaginal 88, 89
sweat glands 96

sympathetic system 132–33
synapses 131
synovial fluid 120
syphilis 80, 163
systolic blood pressure 28, 29,
    30, 31

T

tags, skin 99
talking therapies 141
tanning beds 159
T cells 52, 53
tears 100
teeth 64, 65,
    116–17
  caring for **146**
  dental checks **118–19**
temporal lobes 139
tendons 122, 124
testicles (testes) 78, 79
  checking **82**
testosterone 79, 172
tetanus 45
thalassaemia 55
thoracic vertebrae 120
thyroid 32
  function 61
  scanning **171**
tobacco 150, **151**
toenails 158
tongue 116, 138
tonometry 109
tooth decay 117, 118
torso flexor/extensor endurance
    127
touch receptors 138
tourniquets 54
toxins 53
trachea 42, 116
transducer 41
transthoracic scans 39
transversus abdominis 126
travel vaccinations **144**
treadmills 36, 37,
    51, 125
tread patterns 125
triceps 122
trichomoniasis 80

triglycerides 58, 59
tubules 72, 73
tumour marker
    tests **170–71**
Turner's syndrome 174
tympanogram 114–15
tympanometry **114–15**
typhoid 144

U

ulcers
  mouth 119
  stomach 65, 68
ultrasound
  abdominal **70**
  abdominal aortic aneurysm
    scan 40–41, 176
  breast 95, 172
  carotid artery Doppler scan
    169
  echocardiography 27, 39
  pelvic 85, 90
  testicles 82
ultraviolet light 97, 99,
    159, 161
underweight 24
units of alcohol 150
urea 69, 77
ureters 72
urethra 72, 78, 83
  urethral swab
    test 81
urinary tract infections (UTI) 74,
    75
urine
  analysis **74–75**
  kidney function **76–77**
  nervous system 133
  pregnancy tests 85, **87**
  prostate enlargement 83
  regulation 73
  samples 74
  STIs 81, 88, 89
  urinary system **72–73**
urobilinogen 75
urticaria 99
uterus 84, 85, 86, 93
UTI *see* urinary tract infections

V

vaccinations 17, 81, 88,
   144-45, 160
   records 178-79
vagina 7, 84,
   85, 90
   cervical screening 92
   vaginal swabs
      88, 89
Valsalva manoeuvre 174
valves
   heart 26, 39
   veins 27
varicoceles 82
vas deferens 78,
   79, 82
veins 26, 27, 54
ventilation 42
ventricles 26, 28
vertebrae 120,
   130, 131
veruccas 99,
   158
vestibular nerve 111
vestibular system 111
vibrations 110,
   111
   vibration sensation 137
villi 65
viral infections 80,
   144
vision **100-109**, **177**
vision and memory
   area 138
visual association
   cortex 139
visual field 101,
   108
vitamins
   blood tests 61
   in diet 146, 147, 161
   pregnancy 87
   vitamin D 97, 156,
      157, 158
volume 112, 113
vulva 84

W

waist size 21, 24
walking
   gait **125**
   tests 51
warts 99, 158
   genital 80
waste removal 26,
   42
   role of blood 52
   role of kidneys
      72-73
water
   in diet 146
   safe 12
   in urine 76
wax, ear 110,
   114, 160
weight
   and alcohol 150
   and bone
      health 156
   and breathing 47
   and cholesterol 59
   and diet 148
   and fertility 163
   and health 13,
      24-25
   and heart 34
   home monitoring 21
   keeping fit 153
   and kidneys 77
   records 180
   and skin 158
weight-bearing
   exercises 157
Wernicke's area 138
white blood cells 52, 53,
   55, 75
womb see uterus
working
   memory 139
workplace
   health checks **17**,
      178
   healthy 12
wrist pulse 32

XYZ

X-rays
   angiography 170
   chest 43, **44**
   CT scans 169
   dental 117, 118
   DEXA scan 173
   digestive system 65
   mammography **95**
   musculoskeletal
      system 122
yeast 75
yellow fever 144

Acknowledgments

Dorling Kindersley would like to thank the following people for their assistance in preparing this book: Dr Shannon Hach for checking the contents; Dr Max Balm for his advice on some of the medical tests; Lori Cates Hand, Barbara Campbell, and Bethany Patch for regional information; Michael Clark for editorial assistance; Katy Smith for design assistance; Ann Baggaley and Jamie Ambrose for proofreading; Helen Peters for the index; and Rakesh Kumar (DTP Designer), Priyanka Sharma (Jackets Editorial Coordinator), and Saloni Singh (Managing Jackets Editor).

DK India would like to thank George Thomas for design assistance; Neeraj Bhatia for technical assistance; and Aditya Katyal for picture research assistance.

The publisher would like to thank the following for their kind permission to reproduce their photographs:

(Key: a-above; b-below/bottom; c-centre; f-far; l-left; r-right; t-top)

6-7 iStockphoto.com: E+ / filadendron. **33 iStockphoto.com:** E+ / kali9. **35 Alamy Stock Photo:** Burger / Phanie (b). **36 Getty Images:** Westend61. **iStockphoto.com:** E+ / andresr (cra). **38 Alamy Stock Photo:** APHP-PSL-GARO / Phanie (b). **39 Science Photo Library:** Aberration Films Ltd (t). **40-41 iStockphoto.com:** E+ / andresr (t). **44 Dreamstime.com:** Tyler Olson (b); Rattanachot2525 (cra). **45 Alamy Stock Photo:** Science Photo Library / Ian Hooton (cr). **46 Alamy Stock Photo:** Burger / Phanie. **49 Alamy Stock Photo:** Garo / Phanie (t). **50 Alamy Stock Photo:** Burger / Phanie (b). **51 iStockphoto.com:** E+ / Photomick (cb). **54 Alamy Stock Photo:** BSIP SA / B. Boissonnet (b). **60 Alamy Stock Photo:** Science Photo Library / Tek Image. **63 123RF.com:** belchonock (cr). **Alamy Stock Photo:** Science Photo Library (crb). **66 Science Photo Library:** James King-Holmes (t). **68 Science Photo Library** (t). **70 Getty Images:** DigitalVision / kuniharu wakabayashi (b). **71 Getty Images:** The Image Bank / Lester Lefkowitz (cr). **74 Dreamstime.com:** Jovanmandic (b). **75 Dreamstime.com:** Xannondale (cla). **77 Dreamstime.com:** Ali Rıza Yıldız (r). **80-81 Dreamstime.com:** Sarinya Pinngam (t). **89 Alamy Stock Photo:** Fredrick Kippe (r). **Dreamstime.com:** Henrik Dolle (bl). **93 Alamy Stock Photo:** Westend61 GmbH / Christian Vorhofer (tl). **Dreamstime.com:** Ilexx (tr). **95 iStockphoto.com:** E+ / pixelfit (t). **98 Alamy Stock Photo:** Science Photo Library (r). **Science Photo Library:** Dr P. Marazzi (clb). **99 Alamy Stock Photo:** Mediscan (cl). **103 Dreamstime.com:** Arne9001 (t). **104 Science Photo Library:** Mark Thomas (bl). **105 Dreamstime.com:** Eveleen007 (r). **106-107 Alamy Stock Photo:** Mehmet Çetin (b). **107 Getty Images:** Photodisc / Andrew Dernie (cla); Photodisc / Jacobs Stock Photography (crb). **109 Science Photo Library:** Ralph Eagle (br). **112 iStockphoto.com:** kentarus (cr). **114 Alamy Stock Photo:** BSIP SA / Mendil (cr). **118-119 Dreamstime.com:** Denys Kovtun (t). **118 Alamy Stock Photo:** Science Photo Library (bl). **128 iStockphoto.com:** ruizluquepaz (tr). **129 Dreamstime.com:** Hootie2710 (b). **134 iStockphoto.com:** Jan-Otto (tr). **135 Dreamstime.com:** Wavebreakmedia Ltd (t). **Science Photo Library:** Oxford University Images (b). **141 Alamy Stock Photo:** Burger / Phanie (tr). **146 iStockphoto.com:** E+ / laflor (br). **151 Alamy Stock Photo:** BSIP SA / B. Boissonnet (t). **Dreamstime.com:** Gawriloff (br). **153 Alamy Stock Photo:** Cultura Creative (RF) / Eugenio Marongiu (b). **154 Getty Images:** DigitalVision / Taiyou Nomachi (b). **155 iStockphoto.com:** E+ / PeopleImages (tr). **157 iStockphoto.com:** E+ / gilaxia (t). **159 Alamy Stock Photo:** Paik Photography (br). **Dreamstime.com:** Paultarasenko (t). **160 Getty Images:** Creativ Studio Heinemann (cr). **161 Getty Images:** Moment / MirageC (cra); The Image Bank / Catherine Delahaye (bl). **162 iStockphoto.com:** KatarzynaBialasiewicz (b). **163 Getty Images:** Science Photo Library (tr). **iStockphoto.com:** Napadon Srisawang (clb). **164-165 Dreamstime.com:** Lightfieldstudiosprod (t). **168 Science Photo Library:** Sovereign, ISM. **172 Science Photo Library:** James King-Holmes (tl, ca). **173 Science Photo Library:** James Cavallini (tl). **175 SuperStock:** Phanie / Phanie (tr)

All other images © Dorling Kindersley

For further information see: www.dkimages.com